P9-BBV-123

Overcoming Postpartum Depression & Anxiety

LINDA SEBASTIAN

Addicus Books, Inc.
Omaha, Nebraska

Property of
Lodi Memorial Library

ADG-3349
618.76
SEB

An Addicus Nonfiction Book

Copyright 1998 by Linda Sebastian. All rights reserved. No part of this publication may be reproduced, stored in a retrieval system, or transmitted in any form or by any means electronic, mechanical, photocopied, recorded, or otherwise, without the prior written permission of the publisher. For information, write Addicus Books, Inc., P.O. Box 45327, Omaha, Nebraska 68145.

ISBN 1-886039-30-5

Cover design by Jeff Reiner
Typography by Linda Dageforde
Neuron illustration by Bob Hogenmiller

This book is not intended to serve as a substitute for a physician, nor does the author intend to give medical advice contrary to that of an attending physician.

Library of Congress Cataloging-in-Publication Data

Sebastian, Linda, 1949-
    Overcoming postpartum depression and anxiety / by Linda Sebastian.
        p.   cm.
    Includes bibliographical references and index.
    ISBN 1-886039-34-8 (pbk. : alk. paper)
    1. Postpartum depression. 2. Anxiety in women. I. Title.
RG852.S43 1998   98-16262
618.7'6 — dc21   CIP

LODI MEMORIAL LIBRARY, NJ
3 9139 05069022 2

Addicus Books, Inc.
P.O. Box 45327
Omaha, Nebraska 68145
Web site: http://members.aol.com/addicusbks

Printed in the United States of America
10 9 8 7 6 5 4 3 2

*To the women and their families
with whom I've been privileged to work*

CONTENTS

v

Acknowledgments

I wish to extend a special thanks to Tom Averill; Meredith Titus, Ph.D.; Elizabeth Davis; Jeff Ostergren; and especially Canda Byrne, A.R.N.P., who hung in there with me from start to finish. Thanks to Lee Cohen, M.D., for his pioneering work in the field of perinatal psychiatry and for his encouragement, and Martin Maldonado, M.D.; Robert Barnett, M.D.; Grace Morrison, M.D.; and Breck Edds, M.D., for sharing their perspectives and contributing to this book.

I thank Manya Schmidt, C.N.M., A.R.N.P., for her contributions and her guidance, and Joyce Venis, R.N., of Depression after Delivery for her contributions. I am also grateful to the Menninger Writers Group for their helpful comments, encouragement, and especially writing comradeship. A special thanks goes to Mary Ann Clifft, Director of Scientific Publications at Menninger, for her guidance and editing.

To Kathryn Zerbe, M.D.; Harriet Lerner, Ph.D.; and Glen Gabbard, M.D., many thanks for sharing your wisdom. To the staff at the Professional Library at Menninger...your help was invaluable to me.

Finally, I thank my family—my daughter Rene Almeling for her editing, research, and general giddiness about this project, my son David Almeling for his support, contributions, and the encouraging card at a time when I really needed it, and especially my husband, Guy Almeling, for his considerable faith in me, for making sure my computer was working, and for his persistent encouragement.

Introduction

Like most new mothers or mothers-to-be, you probably have heard of postpartum depression. But, you probably thought that it happened to other women, and would never happen to you. That's what I thought, too. During my first pregnancy, I viewed motherhood as a blissful and perfect time. But, after the birth of my first child, I found myself crying for no reason several times a day. Irritable and cranky, I often found myself in tears over the slightest problem. Because I could not determine why I was crying, I was constantly worried. I felt totally inadequate as a mother. Shame and fear that I was not going to be able to cope with this new person in my life overwhelmed me.

I had read all the pregnancy and new mother books, never imagining *I* would have such a reaction. After all, I had wanted this baby very much. So even though I *thought* I was prepared, I was caught off guard by the roller coaster of my moods. This scary time lasted two weeks before I began to feel better.

Fortunately, I had an understanding and helpful partner who took over the care of the baby when he got home at night so I could rest. I thought I was letting him down by not being a better mother for our new baby. A neighbor who had several children helped me through this time by assuring me that I was not going crazy, that this was "normal," and that I would get over it. Her advice was simple: get as much sleep as you can and tell company not to visit for awhile. She did not tell me not to cry, or ask me why I was crying. This kind neighbor's acceptance was *so* helpful. I don't know what I would have done without her.

Our society does not prepare the new mother and her partner for the overwhelming adjustment to parenthood. The childbirth classes we took emphasized only how to prepare for the big event: labor and delivery. We learned all about breathing and stages of labor. But there was little discussion about the adjustment period following the birth and no mention of how devastating postpartum blues can be, let alone the possibility of more severe depression. The myth that mothers instinctively love their children and always enjoy being mothers only increases the risk of problems for women. It does not prepare them for reality.

As a nurse, I have worked with women who experienced unexpected mood changes or uncomfortable tension after the birth of their babies. As a psychotherapist, I have seen many women and their families suffer from the effects of depression and anxiety. The lack of information only worsens the situation. Often, neither health care professionals nor the public have ready access to information about the emotional problems that occur after childbirth. As you will read, there are many reasons for this lack of information.

This book is for women who are experiencing mood changes or anxiety after delivery. It provides the kind of information that would have been helpful to me when, as a new mother, I thought I was going crazy.

*The only thing that seems eternal and natural
in motherhood is ambivalence.*

—Jane Lazarre
Novelist

1

The Unexpected and Unknown

I was so excited about this baby. We had waited four years after we were married and saved our money, so I didn't have to go back to work. I worried about the baby having all its parts or being healthy, but I didn't worry about me. When I couldn't stop crying after I got home with the baby, I was so scared and thought I was a terrible mother. No one told me this might happen.

Annette, 32-year-old mother

Annette's anticipation of the birth of her child is very common. Most women expect an uneventful pregnancy and delivery. If anything, women usually worry more about the health of their babies than about their own health. For the majority of women, this time in their lives is, indeed, healthy. However, many women experience problems with depression and anxiety both during their pregnancy and after delivery. Because information about the potential emotional complications after childbirth is usually not shared with women, those who do have these problems often feel alone and isolated.

Postpartum depression describes a spectrum of mood disorders that typically occur in about 1 in 10 women after delivery. These mood disorders range from *postpartum blues* on the mild end of the spectrum to *postpartum major depression, postpartum anxiety disorders*, and *postpartum psychotic depression* on the more severe end of the spectrum. Such illnesses can devastate a woman and her family, as well as affect her newborn.

A majority (60 to 80 percent) of all women who bear children experience milder problems, such as postpartum blues. About 10 to 15 percent of women who have a baby will develop major depression or severe anxiety. Only a small percentage (about 1 in 1,000) develops the more severe psychotic depression.

Just as most women who suffer from major depression also have some anxiety, women with anxiety disorders usually experience some depression. There is a strong connection between anxiety and depression. Usually these problems occur together. These disorders are covered separately later in this book to help you clearly understand the symptoms.

Why is this problem misunderstood?

You may be unclear about postpartum mood disorders as a result of the terms used to describe them. The term *postpartum depression* is commonly used to describe the whole range of emotional problems surrounding childbirth. A majority of women know about the mild form called *postpartum blues*, which is often erroneously referred to as postpartum depression. The more serious forms of depression and anxiety that require professional help are also labeled postpartum depression. This overlapping language only creates confusion among women and their families, as well as health care professionals unfamiliar with psychiatric problems. The lack of clarity may cause the more severe problems to be confused with the less severe postpartum blues. Since the more severe problems are not recognized, they often go untreated.

To promote clarity, this book uses the specific terms *postpartum blues*, *postpartum depression*, *postpartum psychosis*, and *postpartum anxiety* rather than the more generic *postpartum depression*. When a general term is required, the phrase *postpartum mood disorders* is used. Since postpartum mood disorders have different symptoms, different treatments, and possibly different causes, it is important to discuss each one separately. Bear in mind, however, that sometimes the problems overlap and may be difficult to distinguish from one another. For example, in the second- or third-week postpartum, it may be difficult to tell if you are experiencing postpartum blues or postpartum depression. For this reason, it is important to consult a mental health professional as soon as you notice problems.

Two secondary factors also contribute to the lack of information about postpartum mood disorders. First, in today's smaller families, women usually have little experience caring for the babies of others or being around women who are having babies. Their lack of experience, coupled with unrealistic expectations, increases their fear of inadequacy. Many women have never known anyone else who had depression or anxiety after delivery. Because there is a stigma associated with psychiatric disorders in our society, women do not tell other women what has happened to them. This may contribute to the lack of information about risk factors for these problems. Second, extended families usually live too far away to help at home during the crucial first two weeks after delivery. Many working women who give birth feel alone because both their peer and social groups remain at work or their families are unavailable. Having a baby separates a woman from her support system and keeps her isolated at home. As you will discover later in this book, this isolation may contribute to mood disorders.

Culturally, our society pays a lot of attention to women and their partners during pregnancy and delivery. There is an expectation that all will be well after delivery. The mother should go home to do what comes naturally: take care of her baby without help or guidance. However, more attention should be paid to the new mother and her mental health. The postpartum period is the time of highest risk for a woman to be hospitalized with a psychiatric disorder.

Compounding the confusion for new mothers and their families is health care professionals' lack of awareness about these disorders. The major obstetric and gynecologic texts in use today, like those of the past forty years, generally do not mention the risk of postpartum mood disorders. If they do, it is only briefly. They neither list the risk factors nor provide a guide to treatment. As a result of this oversight, nurses and physicians who work with pregnant women and their families are not consistently assessing women for mood disorders.

There does not seem to be a clear reason for this oversight in the training of health care practitioners. Dr. Robert Barnett, an obstetrician and gynecologist in the Midwest, describes his experience in his residency program:

> *We were taught almost nothing about psychiatric disorders related to pregnancy and delivery. In my residency, the emphasis was on illness or problems related to*

gynecology or obstetrics. In four years of medical school, we probably received about one hour of lecture on psychiatric problems.

Dr. Grace Morrison, another Midwestern obstetrician, proposes that postpartum disorders are not well-known because women's problems have often been overlooked in medicine. Most of the research, treatment guidelines, and medical and nursing training has been conducted on or about men. Another possible reason for the oversight is the medicalization of childbirth, according to Manya Schmidt, a certified nurse-midwife in Kansas:

> *Childbirth was brought into the hospital, and women were taken away from their families. The entire pregnancy and after delivery was once a midwife's domain. What was once a natural event became a medical event with little attention paid to the woman after delivery.*

The consequences of this lack of medical training is clear. It means that no one may be educating you or your partner about these risks. No one may recognize these serious problems when they occur.

Childbirth preparation classes often prepare women for the *physical* complications of delivery—infection and hemorrhage—but many never mention the possibility of postpartum disorders. Yet the incidence of postpartum depression is greater than the incidence of either of these other two potential complications. The rate of postpartum infection after a vaginal delivery is about 3 percent. As stated previously, the estimated rate of severe postpartum depression is about 10 percent.

Furthermore, our health care system divides our bodies into physical and mental parts. This specialization encourages health care professionals to know only one part of the body well. For all intents and purposes, they are ignorant about the rest of the body. When illnesses like postpartum mood disorders involve both psychological and physical aspects, the problems often do not fall within a health care specialist's domain. So often the problems go unrecognized and untreated.

The tragedy inherent in the unclear language, the lack of information for health care professionals, and the compartmentalization of health care means that we cannot identify who is most at risk for developing postpartum problems. Even though postpartum depression is one of the few mental health problems for which we can predict who is most at risk, many women do not receive the treatment they need to prevent more serious problems. Additionally, many women receive treatment only when symptoms get so severe that they are unmanageable. This means that it takes longer for the symptoms to subside.

Are postpartum mood disorders a new problem?

Since the time of Hippocrates, we have known that mothers can experience problems with their mood after delivery. The first medically documented study of emotional disorders after childbirth was in 1838 by a French physician, Dr. Jean E. Esquirol. Another French physician, Louis Marcé, continued to study these disorders and wrote extensively about them in the mid-1800s. Marcé delineated three kinds of problems related to the postpartum period: problems first seen in pregnancy, those seen immediately after delivery, and those seen about six weeks after delivery. His pioneering work helped clinicians recognize that there is more than one kind of psychiatric problem related to pregnancy and childbirth.

Marcé's work is still viewed today as the first attempt to categorize postpartum psychiatric disorders. Marcé also believed that problems in the postpartum period were unique to this time in a woman's life, distinct from psychiatric problems outside the postpartum period. The Marcé Society, an international organization devoted to the study and treatment of postpartum disorders, is named in his honor. It is a major source of information and collaboration about postpartum psychiatric disorders worldwide.

After Marcé's work, there was little investigation of postpartum psychiatric problems until the 1980s. In the 1920s, psychiatrists who developed a classification system for psychiatric disorders left out postpartum mood disorders because they did not consider them distinct from other psychiatric disorders. As a result, generations of psychiatric professionals such as psychiatrists, psychiatric nurses, psychologists, and social workers are not fully aware of the psychiatric risks accompanying childbirth.

Yet postpartum problems are among the few psychiatric disorders that mental health professionals have been successful in preventing, or at least in modifying their severity. There is still debate, however, as to whether postpartum disorders are unique to this time period or are similar to depression and anxiety found in both men and women at other times in their lives. In one British study, women who had gynecologic surgery were compared to women who had delivered a baby. A questionnaire examined their mood changes. Significant differences between the two groups of women support the idea that postpartum mood changes are unique to childbirth.

Just as postpartum disorders were found in ancient civilizations, they are found worldwide today. Women in both industrialized countries and "undeveloped" countries demonstrate an increased risk of hospitalization for psychiatric reasons after childbirth.

Who is at risk for developing anxiety and depression?

If you have previously suffered postpartum depression or other episodes of depression or anxiety, you are among the most likely to develop problems with the birth of a child. You are also at risk if you have experienced severe postpartum blues or have had mood changes related to your menstrual cycle. Another risk factor is major stress or change during pregnancy, such as a move, a death in the family, conflict with a spouse or partner, or potential problems with the unborn baby. Problems during delivery, either with the baby or the mother, also increase the risk of mood disorders after delivery. Other risk factors include social isolation after the mother and baby are home and a lack of supportive family members who actually help with the housework and help care for the baby.

Two significant risk factors for depression are childhood abuse and trauma. Sexual abuse, physical abuse, neglect, and overwhelming traumatic experiences such as the loss of a parent or sibling place women at risk for depression and anxiety even without the added stress of pregnancy and mothering.

To detect women at risk and refer them to appropriate psychiatric professionals, obstetricians and nurse-midwives could easily ask a few questions about the mental health history of the soon-to-be-pregnant woman or expectant mother. Questions about the stress levels in the woman's life—especially about the quality of her marital relationship—are just as important as questions about physical symptoms, to which Lisa's story attests:

> *When I was pregnant the first time, we had just moved to a new town, and my father had died. I was stressed during my pregnancy and was very depressed after the baby came, but I never told anyone or got any help. No one asked about my mental state.*
>
> *This time, I was asked about stress in my pregnancy and previous depression. I was told I was at risk and was referred to a therapist in the third trimester. I was so relieved to have someone recognize that I needed psychological help as well as monitoring of my pregnancy. Things went much better because I had emotional help and support.*

As a psychotherapist, in my own work I provide a list of symptoms and screening questions to obstetric nurses and physicians. They are now better able to detect potential and actual cases of postpartum depression, resulting in preventive action or early treatment in many cases.

In addition to the lack of awareness of these problems, our society minimizes the impact of having a baby, especially a first baby. Recently, "drive-through deliveries" have gained widespread attention in the media and even in the U.S. Congress. Insurance companies, managed care companies, and other third-party payers want to reduce costs, so they require the hospital stay to be as brief as possible. In other words, this trend reflects the attitude that having a baby is "no big deal" and that a woman should quickly return home to carry on with her life. But, in fact, the physiological and psychological changes that you experience at delivery are unparalleled in your entire life.

What can I expect to feel if I have postpartum problems?

When depression or anxiety affects you as a new mother in the postpartum period, you may not realize what is happening. You might think fatigue is making you feel unable to care for your baby, or you might think your hormones are making you "jittery." Because all of us are different, it is impossible to predict exactly how you are going to feel or react to having a baby. Most women report tearfulness as a primary concern, but for others it is irritability.

For most women, as symptoms worsen, they often try to hide their problems and avoid contact with others. Unaware that other women share her problem, they feel alone. They believe they are "bad" mothers to be having the feelings that accompany postpartum depression. Isolation, guilt, and shame worsen this depression. Tragically, this situation is all too common, but it is one that can often be prevented. If new mothers and their families realize that depression and anxiety are possible, they may seek early treatment before the symptoms worsen.

What influence does weaning the baby have?

If you are having mood changes and do not feel as well as you think you should, weaning the baby may seem like a solution. In fact, for some women, a stop to breast-feeding improves their mood because they are likely to get more rest and may return to a more stable, pre-pregnant state. Some women notice no difference in their mood upon weaning the baby. However, other women experience mood changes only when they stop breast-feeding. If mood changes occur during weaning, it is likely that a woman will experience similar problems with weaning after future deliveries. Consider the story of Paulette, a twenty-eight-year-old mother of two.

> *I noticed that I became very depressed for about one month after I stopped nursing my first baby. I cried for no reason, couldn't sleep, and generally felt miserable. I thought it was because I missed nursing.*
>
> *With my second baby, it happened again. I was working then as a nurse. Nursing was a stress and a strain, and I didn't want to do it. When I got very depressed again, to the point where I could not get out of bed or take care of my kids, I knew I needed help.*

It is believed that changes in the level of prolactin, a hormone present in high levels during breastfeeding, may be responsible for mood changes related to weaning. If you are having problems with your mood, consult a mental health professional before attempting to wean on your own.

Are all postpartum problems alike?

Dr. Deborah Sichel, an east coast psychiatrist and researcher, is one of the clinicians continuing Marcé's work. She proposes that there are six categories of women who suffer postpartum problems.

She characterizes one group as a "pure" group. These women experience an early, severe onset of symptoms and have problems only after delivery. This group is also likely to have emotional problems after each delivery.

Sichel's second group includes women with a previous history of depression or *dysthymia*, a mild form of depression. These women may or may not have been previously diagnosed or treated. They are at risk of mood changes both during pregnancy and after delivery.

Her third group is women who primarily suffer anxiety, not depression. Often these women have had a high degree of anxiety for most of their adult lives. This anxiety worsens after delivery.

The fourth group is composed of women who get depressed during pregnancy. Often the first onset of depression is during their first trimester. Usually their depression worsens as the pregnancy continues.

Sichel's fifth group is women who have a kind of mood disorder called *manic-depressive illness* or *bipolar disorder*. These women typically have a history of ups and downs. The postpartum episode of mood swings is usually very severe and may include psychotic symptoms.

The sixth and last group are women who have postpartum blues. It is believed that about 25 percent of these women will develop a more severe form of depression later in life.

Another leading researcher who continues the work of Marcé is Dr. Lee Cohen, director of Perinatal Psychiatry at Massachusetts General Hospital. Cohen's studies have helped debunk the myth that women with anxiety disorders have fewer symptoms during pregnancy as a result of elevated estrogen levels. Unfortunately, this myth—even among health professionals—has led to many women's problems being minimized. Cohen did what is considered the first "prospective" study. (Most studies are "retrospective" or looking back.) Cohen studied women with anxiety disorders as they went through their pregnancies. He concluded that their level of anxiety continued to be high, that pregnancy does not offer protection against anxiety and depression.

As we have seen, a hundred years after the groundbreaking work of Marcé, the psychiatric community once again recognizes that women may suffer from, and families may be affected by, postpartum mood disorders. Controversy continues about whether the illnesses of the postpartum period are unique to that time or whether the depression and anxiety are identical to those experienced at other times. Although there are many unanswered questions about the problems women have after childbirth, we do know how to help. Gathering information is the first step you can take toward feeling better and mastering the bewildering changes after delivery.

2

The Roller Coaster of Postpartum Blues

Maternity blues, baby blues, natal blues, and postpartum blues are all terms used to describe the temporary tearfulness, mood swings, fatigue, and irritability that you might experience in the first two weeks after giving birth. This reaction is so common that it is considered "normal," even though the woman experiencing maternity blues does not feel normal at all. Paula, a twenty-four-year-old mother, recalls her experience after giving birth:

> *When I got home from the hospital, I was so happy I was giddy. My baby was perfect. Labor was not as bad as I thought it would be. The first day I was home, I burst into tears. I couldn't figure out why I was crying. Then I would be ecstatic again. This roller coaster scared me because I could never predict how I was going to feel. I thought I was the only one who ever cried after having a new baby at home. Finally, after ten days, I stopped the crying and began to feel good about myself and the baby.*

When do the blues start?

Postpartum blues usually begin one or two days after delivery and last two to three weeks. The symptoms of true postpartum blues will subside if they do not mark the beginning of severe depression, and you will soon begin to feel more like your old self. During these first two weeks, it is difficult to distinguish between depression and the blues. If you have not had a previous depression and if the symptoms are not severe, the health care professionals working with you may want to wait to gauge the severity and longevity of your blues before beginning treatment.

Women who have the blues describe themselves on a "mood roller coaster." They feel euphoric and elated, then their mood plummets to despondency and anxiety. This frightening, out-of-control feeling adds to their anxiety and fear. Some women understand this pattern of extreme mood swings as a normal reaction to the tremendous physical and psychological upheaval of having a baby. For others, the symptoms translate into a suggestion that they are not good mothers, so they fear they are *never* going to be good mothers. Many women also worry that their behavior will affect the baby. The unexpectedness of these feelings adds to the feeling of being out of control.

What causes postpartum blues?

Although the cause of the blues is not completely understood, the main contributors are probably the changes in your body related to childbirth, the fatigue of caring for a new baby, and the monumental adjustment of becoming a mother.

The physical changes in your body as you undergo labor and delivery are unparalleled. At no other time in adulthood does the female body experience such a tremendous upheaval. The change in hormone levels from pregnancy to postdelivery is drastic. The stress response to labor and delivery alone can lead to a "letdown" and shaky sensation. Blood volume, blood pressure, changes in the immune system, and changes in metabolism are just a few of the many changes your body undergoes.

The major psychological change that occurs as you adjust to motherhood is also unprecedented. The abruptness of the change in becoming a parent may be one factor that contributes to maternity blues. Even though the nine-month pregnancy is a preparation of sorts, there is no way to prepare either you or your partner for the awesome and overwhelming responsibility of having a child.

Compounding the physical and psychological changes is fatigue. If you had major surgery or had been injured in a car accident with resulting physical damages, you would be put to bed for rest. But women are expected to have a baby and not skip a step. Because childbirth is a "natural" event, it is perceived that the changes will have little impact. Yet the physical and psychological changes of pregnancy and childbirth are in themselves exhausting and overwhelming. Add to that mix the lack of sleep that accompanies having a newborn, and there is sufficient reason why you might be on an emotional roller coaster! *Nevertheless, fatigue is often underplayed as a major contributing factor in postpartum blues.* Several factors may combine to make you feel overly fatigued: visitors, early discharge from the hospital (often after being there only a few hours), lack of support from the extended family, lack of paternity leave for fathers, and the minimization in our culture of the childbirth event itself.

What are the risk factors for postpartum blues?

The biggest predictor of postpartum blues seems to be a previous episode of the blues. If you had postpartum blues once, then you are at high risk for another episode. The relationship of other mood disorders to postpartum blues is not so clear-cut. Some professionals believe there is no relationship between postpartum blues and a previous psychiatric history. However, a study by Dr. Michael O'Hara, past president of the Marcé Society, reports an increased risk for postpartum blues among women with depression during pregnancy, with at least one previous episode of depression in their lives, with higher levels of premenstrual depression, or with a close blood relative with a mood disorder. These conflicting results probably reflect the lack of a clear definition for the blues and the lack of a consistently valid measurement tool. Predicting who is most at risk for postpartum blues remains unclear.

If this is your first baby and you have one or more of these risk factors, discuss the possibility that you might have the emotional ups and downs of postpartum blues with your family. Also, be sure to discuss your history with your health care provider.

What should you do if you have postpartum blues?

First, as I mentioned earlier, recognize that *most* women experience the blues. Your tears, your elation, your fatigue, and your worries are all part of a normal adjustment process to one of the biggest changes you will ever experience. Paula, the new mother you met at the beginning of the chapter, continues:

The experience of having the mood changes was bad enough, but I thought it meant that I had made a big mistake by wanting to be a mother. I thought all mothers who really wanted their babies were happy. Since I wasn't completely happy, I assumed I wasn't meant to be a mother.

It is very important not to assign a negative meaning to your symptoms as Paula did. If you assume that you are having these feelings because you are not a good mother, or because you are weak, or because you do not really want a baby, you may actually increase the severity of your symptoms and the length of time it takes to adjust to the physical changes and your new role. But if you tell yourself that your reaction is very typical of new mothers and that it is signaling you to get some rest and pamper yourself, then your recovery will probably be faster. Our body believes what we tell it: tell yours good things.

Getting plenty of rest is the single most important thing you can do. Many new mothers downplay this advice and think, "Other women don't need this much rest," or "I shouldn't have to spend so much time resting. After all, childbirth is a natural process." Sleep is required to heal physically, to adjust psychologically, to make milk, and to stabilize your mood. We can drastically alter the mood of healthy people who have not experienced massive physical changes simply by depriving them of sleep. Terrorists know that they can make their prisoners lose touch with reality if they keep them awake long enough. Why, then, do new mothers assume they are immune to this phenomenon?

In addition to sleep, your other physical needs must be fulfilled, including eating well and drinking plenty of liquids. This logical advice often goes unsaid. However, many women ignore cues from their body about the need for food and drink because of the changes in their bodies, their disrupted sleep schedules, or simply because they think they have no good reason to feel fatigued.

If you find yourself crying and are not able to identify a reason for your weeping, stop looking for one. You do not need a reason to cry, but you can use the tearfulness and anxiety as a signal that you do need more sleep. Everyone has individual needs. Pay attention to yours. Sleep while the baby sleeps. If you need to ask for some help with the baby so you can get more sleep, then do so. To sleep soundly for a few hours, you may even need to get away from the baby. If doing so will help you rest better, make arrangements for the baby to leave the house so you can relax and sleep. Your baby will benefit from *your* rest.

The time immediately after childbirth is *not* the time to tackle home projects like cleaning closets, painting the living room, or doing other things you have been wanting to do once you were at home for awhile. Joy, a thirty-one-year-old first-time mother, remembers her experience well.

> *My friends and family warned me that I was not going to be able to keep the house as clean as I liked once the baby got here, but I didn't believe them. I had always been efficient and kept the house very neat. I was sure I would be able to handle everything. I planned on painting most of the house inside when I was home on maternity leave. As you can imagine, I had to adjust to a new standard of housekeeping, and the house did not get painted!*

Tell people who want to visit to wait a few weeks until you and the baby have adjusted to your new routine. If it is hard for you to say no, then use an answering machine to screen calls or allow your helpers to do that for you. If people offer to help, ask them to bring a meal or to come over to dust and vacuum the living room. People like to feel helpful and appreciate concrete suggestions.

If your friends or relatives are not coming to see you (because they think you want to be left alone) and you need to see some familiar faces or talk to friends, call them. Tell them you are going stir-crazy and ask them to come see you and bring all the latest news.

This is a time to "baby" yourself. Doing so may be difficult because you are so focused on your baby. But remember, your baby needs you to be healthy and at your best. Our society teaches women to put other people's needs before our own. If this is your pattern, think of a balance between your needs and those of the baby. If you need to get out of the house for a change of scenery, your baby will do just fine with someone else for a few hours. If you are having trouble getting enough sleep, perhaps your partner can do the last feeding and put the baby to bed. You will get a better start on a good night's sleep, and the two of them will begin to bond. Remember that you, too, are a person with needs, not just a mother.

If your moodiness does not seem to improve or if you are unable to sleep while the baby is asleep, then you should seek professional help. If you are feeling desperate and fear you cannot continue feeling as you do, call someone immediately. Don't wait a week or two to see if you will start to feel better. At the very least, you will probably experience some relief in talking with someone about how you feel. You will also get an objective opinion and may begin treatment if it is needed.

3

Postpartum Anxiety Disorders

To understand the various kinds of *anxiety disorders* that may accompany pregnancy and the postpartum period, it is helpful for you to first understand the kind of anxiety that nearly everyone experiences. People with anxiety disorders often report that others minimize, or brush off, their problems. This may occur because all people experience anxiety. Most people do not understand the difference between anxiety disorders and normal anxiety.

Anxiety is a part of our lives. It is a normal and protective response to events outside the range of everyday human experience. It helps us concentrate and focus on tasks. It helps us avoid dangerous situations. Anxiety also provides motivation to accomplish things that we may otherwise tend to put off. As you can see, anxiety is essential to our survival.

Anxiety is often described as a spectrum of feelings. Just about everyone experiences mild or moderate anxiety as we go about our work and play. When we have moderate anxiety, our heart rates increase minimally so that there is more oxygen available. We are alert so we can focus better on a task or problem. Our muscles are slightly tensed so we can move and work. Our production of hormones, such as adrenaline and insulin, is slightly elevated to help the body react. We can study for a test, prepare a report for work, give a speech, or hit the ball when we are up to bat. If we were completely relaxed, we could not concentrate or accomplish these tasks. Anxiety helps us meet the demands made on us.

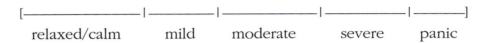

relaxed/calm   mild   moderate   severe   panic

The subjective feeling we call anxiety is accompanied by a predictable pattern of bodily responses summarized in the continuum above. People with anxiety disorders have reactions, designed to help us escape danger, in situations that are *not* life threatening. The normal mechanism for initiating these responses goes awry for reasons we do not fully understand. When we have severe anxiety, we do not think well and cannot solve problems. Production of adrenaline is so high that it causes a sensation of a "pounding" heart, shortness of breath, and extremely tense muscles. We feel a sense of danger or dread. This fear may or may not have a focus. If we were facing a tiger, this level of anxiety would be helpful to us to fight or flee. However, if this level of anxiety occurs without a dangerous stimulus, this response is not helpful. *Anxiety disorders differ from anxiety in general in that the experience or feelings are more intense and last longer.* Anxiety disorders also interfere with the normal functioning of people at work, at play, and in relationships.

When we are faced with real or imagined threats, our brain signals the body that we are in danger. Hormones are released as part of this general alarm call. These hormones produce the following changes:

- the mind is more alert
- blood clotting ability increases, preparing for injury
- heart rate increases and blood pressure rises (there may be a sensation of the heart pounding and a tightness in the chest)
- sweating increases to help cool the body
- blood is diverted to the muscles to help prepare for action (this may lead to a light-headed feeling as well as a tingling in the hands)
- digestion slows down (this may lead to a heavy feeling like a "lump" in the stomach, as well as nausea)
- saliva production decreases (which leads to a dry mouth and a choking sensation)
- breathing rate increases (which may feel like shortness of breath)
- liver releases sugar to provide quick energy (which may feel like a "rush")
- sphincter muscles contract to close the opening of the bowel and bladder
- immune response decreases (useful in the short term to let the body respond to a threat, but over time harmful to our health)
- thinking speeds up
- there is a sensation of fear, a desire to move or take action, and an inability to sit still

Is anxiety normal for new mothers?

All new mothers are somewhat anxious. Being a mother is a new role, a new job, with a new person in your life and new, responsibilities. Anxiety in response to this situation is very common. Pediatricians, obstetricians, and nurses are used to worries, concerns, and questions like yours.

However, for reasons we cannot explain, some mothers have excessive worries and experience a severe level of anxiety. Dori, a new mother, describes her anxiety:

> *I could not sit still or relax at all. My thoughts were racing, and I couldn't focus on anything at all. I worried constantly that something was wrong with the baby or that I would do something wrong. I had never felt this kind of anxiety before, but I didn't know if it was normal for new mothers.*

As with Dori, mothers with severe anxiety have difficulty enjoying their new babies, and they are overly concerned about minor problems. They have unrealistic fears about doing something wrong to hurt the baby. Mothers with severe anxiety cannot relax when there is an opportunity to do so. *Anxiety disorders are often missed in new mothers because of the belief that all new mothers are excessively anxious.* If you find yourself meeting the criteria for any of the anxiety disorders described in this chapter, or if you are very uncomfortable for prolonged periods such as several hours, talk to your health care provider. Take this book with you and share your concerns, because not all health care providers are familiar with the criteria for anxiety disorders.

Why anxiety disorders and panic for some?

Although anxiety is a normal human response to stress, we are not sure why some people have severe anxiety or panic in response to everyday situations. As with depression, there are several theories about why these problems occur.

One theory proposes that some people have a biological tendency toward anxiety. Some people seem to be more sensitive to the effects of the hormones released during anxiety. There may be a genetic link in some disorders. Because the chemicals in the brain that are affected in anxiety are similar to the ones affected during depression, family history is important in determining what kind of disorder is present and what kind of treatment may help.

Another theory proposes that anxiety is a learned response to negative or fearful situations as we grow up. If you were around someone who was fearful, negative, and/or critical when you were a child, you may have developed a long-standing habit of assuming the worst is going to happen or reacting negatively to events. This theory also explains why trauma, an extremely upsetting event, may play a role in the development of anxiety. If you are in an accident, if you see someone die, or if you are attacked, you may have a reaction that marks the beginning of an anxiety disorder. Reactions to stress and loss may also be a factor.

There is probably no *one* single reason why people develop anxiety disorders. Because we are limited in our understanding of how these disorders develop, it is probably not all that helpful to try to figure out how yours started or which family member "gave" you this problem. You will find it more productive to look at how you can respond differently to situations that make you anxious, to modify the physiological response to these situations, and to master your habit of negative thinking.

People with anxiety disorders are often known as "worriers" concerned about control and perfectionism. These can be good traits to have. But when the need for perfectionism or control interferes with your life, an anxiety disorder often develops.

If you find yourself fitting the criteria for a diagnosis of an anxiety disorder, it is important that the possible physical causes of these symptoms be eliminated. Several physical illnesses may cause symptoms similar to these disorders. A basic principle of mental health treatment is to first rule out any physical causes of symptoms. Some of these physical conditions or illnesses are hypoglycemia (low blood sugar), hyperthyroidism (an overactive thyroid), inner ear problems, mitral valve prolapse, hypertension, and some nutritional deficiencies. While the anxiety symptoms caused by these problems affect only a small percentage of people with the symptoms, it is important to first investigate all the possible causes of the symptoms.

What anxiety disorders are common in the postpartum period?

Women with postpartum anxiety disorders experience a spectrum of problems that range in severity from *adjustment disorder* to *generalized anxiety disorder* (GAD) to *obsessive-compulsive disorder* to *panic disorder*. In this chapter, we'll review the symptoms of each disorder, according to the American Psychological Association's *Diagnostic and Statistical Manual of Mental Disorders.*

It's important to note, however, that these anxiety disorders are not unique to the postpartum period. In fact, anxiety disorders are one of the most common psychiatric problems seen by mental health and family practice professionals. Studies show that more women than men suffer anxiety disorders. About 10 per-cent of women in the United States will have an anxiety disorder sometime in their lives, while 5 percent of men will experience these problems.

Adjustment disorder is a reaction to an external stress beyond what is considered typical. It is usually time-limited and responds well to minimal intervention. Many people have difficulty accommodating to changes in their lives such as divorce, job loss, retirement, or other crises.

Twenty-nine-year-old Darla's story is typical of a problem called adjustment disorder. Although it is not specifically an anxiety disor-der, adjustment disorder is in-cluded in this section because anxiety is such a common feature. However, symptoms of depression may be present also.

Are you having any of these symptoms?

- Are you so anxious that you cannot ade-quately care for your baby?
- Are you afraid of hurting yourself or the baby to the extent that you are not sure you can stop yourself?
- Are your compulsive behaviors harmful to the baby?
- Are you so anxious that you cannot eat or sleep?

If so, consult a mental health professional and tell him/her that you require immediate attention.

After my son was born, I felt "revved up" and could not sit down and relax for a min-ute. I felt like there was a motor inside that would not shut off. I just thought it was the excitement of having the baby we had wanted for so long. When I got home from the hospital, I couldn't sleep at all. I got so tired and irri-table that when he cried I wanted to yell, "Shut up!" This only made me feel worse. I was worried I was not going to be able to handle being a mother. I found myself avoiding taking care of my baby. It took me almost two weeks before I could enjoy him.

Darla was referred to a therapist who helped her learn to relax and to not worry so much about minor problems like diaper rash. Darla tended to "catastrophize." Small events took on life-and-death proportions in her thinking. Darla learned to observe herself catastrophizing and to be more objective in her assessment of situations. After several sessions with the therapist, Darla was less anxious, was beginning to enjoy the baby, and was able to sleep when the baby slept.

Symptoms of Adjustment Disorder

- Emotional or behavioral symptoms develop in response to identifiable stressor(s), occurring within three months of the onset of the stressor(s).
- These symptoms or behaviors are shown by either marked distress in excess of what would normally be expected from exposure to the stressor or by significant impairment in social or occupational functions.
- The symptoms are not related to bereavement or grief.
- The symptoms last no more than six months once the stressor has stopped.

What is generalized anxiety disorder?

A more severe form of anxiety is *generalized anxiety disorder* (GAD). This illness is characterized by a persistent anxiety that affects most areas of a person's life. This disorder is accompanied by worries or fears that are out of proportion to the situation. Many people, men and women alike, have this kind of anxiety but never seek treatment. They are known to their friends and families as "worriers."

If a woman with GAD becomes pregnant, she may feel less anxiety during her pregnancy. But she is likely to experience anxiety again after delivery. Since anxiety continues during pregnancy for some women, it is difficult to predict who will experience anxiety during pregnancy. Jill's story is very typical of a new mother with GAD:

> *I have always been a "worrywart" and have been teased about my nervousness since I was a little girl. I felt pretty good during my pregnancy. But after the baby came, I got much worse. I couldn't sleep, and I was always calling the doctor because I thought something was wrong with the baby. I developed horrible muscle spasms in my neck. The pediatrician suggested I see a therapist about my anxiety. I didn't realize that what I had could be helped.*

Jill meets the criteria for a diagnosis of GAD. She saw a therapist who used a cognitive therapy approach to help her become more aware of how her thinking increased her anxiety. Jill realized that she tended to think of things as either "black or white, right or wrong." She also tended to assume the worst in most situations. Jill learned to use relaxation techniques to help her remain calm. She also learned to change her habit of negative thinking. After a brief therapy process, Jill felt less anxious and enjoyed her baby more.

Generalized Anxiety Disorder Criteria

- Excessive anxiety and worry about a number of events or activities, occurring more days than not for at least six months.
- The person finds it difficult to control the worry.
- The anxiety and worry are associated with three or more of the following symptoms:
    - restlessness, feeling "keyed up," or "on edge"
    - being easily fatigued
    - difficulty concentrating or mind going blank
    - irritability
    - muscle tension
    - sleep disturbance (trouble going to sleep or staying asleep)

What is obsessive-compulsive disorder?

Obsessive-compulsive disorder (OCD) is an anxiety disorder that used to be considered rare. Now psychiatric clinicians recognize it is much more common than originally thought. *Obsessive* and *compulsive* are terms sometimes used to depict people who are perfectionistic, require a certain order, or have rigid routines. Although these characteristics may fit many people, these traits are parts of our personalities. The actual criteria for OCD diagnosis include many more serious symptoms. People with the disorder (rather than just the traits) lead disrupted lives.

This anxiety disorder has two components: thoughts and behavior. *Obsessions* are persistent thoughts that intrude upon the person's consciousness. These thoughts are unwelcome, but the affected person feels incapable of controlling them. Examples of obsessions are thoughts about a body part, saying a word over and over, and thoughts of hurting yourself or someone else.

Among postpartum women, these obsessions are frequently about hurting the baby in some manner, like throwing it against a wall or by hitting or stabbing it. In her book,*Shouldn't I Be Happy? Emotional Problems of Pregnant and Postpartum Women*, Dr. Shaila Misri reports that in addition to the obsessive thought of hurting the baby, another obsession is frequent. She describes a theme of obsessing about previously having killed a baby, which may affect women who have terminated an earlier pregnancy. This theme may also be evident in women who have miscarried.

Compulsions are behaviors that are repetitive and ritualistic. Common compulsions are continuous cleaning, rearranging things such as items in kitchen cabinets, or washing hands. The urge to do these things continually is uncomfortable, but the person feels as if stopping is not possible. Common compulsive behaviors in postpartum women with OCD are frequent bathing of the baby or changing its clothes. Nola, a twenty-five-year-old mother, tells of her OCD episode:

> *After I was home for about two weeks, I began having fears about smothering the baby with her pillow. I could not stop the thoughts from happening.*
>
> *I love my daughter so much, and I felt so ashamed of having these awful thoughts.*
>
> *Finally, I called a crisis hotline. They told me I probably had an anxiety problem called OCD. I was so relieved, I cried for several hours. I was started on a medication, and the thoughts stopped. It was like a miracle!*

Nola's story is very typical of persons with OCD. They recognize that their thinking and behavior is "not normal." Women describe a sense of shame and guilt about having these thoughts and behaviors. They often hide from their family and friends their ritualistic behaviors and obsessive thoughts. Nola reports:

> *I'd had obsessions since I was a child, but thought I could control them. I never told anyone because I was afraid they would send me to a psychiatric hospital. I realize now how much of my life I have spent hiding something that was easily treated. I wish I had gotten help earlier so I would not have had such a hard time when my daughter was born.*

Just like Nola, many of these women suffer in silence because they feel so ashamed of having such thoughts. Often the new mother with OCD will go to great lengths to avoid being alone with her baby. Common strategies are to be gone from home all day to places like the library or shopping mall or out to visit friends. Developing complaints of illness to avoid taking care of the baby is also common.

Because OCD is not a psychotic illness, the mother is unlikely to act on her thoughts, so there is little risk to the infant. Nevertheless, the toll on the mother is tremendous. Some women whose children are now in their twenties with children of their own clearly remember the thoughts they had of possibly harming their babies. They still feel guilty decades later.

In order to meet the criteria for a diagnosis of obsessive-compulsive disorder, either compulsions or obsessions can be present. In addition, at some point, the person has recognized that the obsessions or compulsions are excessive or unreasonable. The obsessions or compulsions cause marked distress, are time-consuming, or significantly interfere with the person's normal routine, occupational functions, or usual social activities or relationships.

Symptoms of Obsessive-Compulsive Disorder

Obsessions are defined by:

- recurrent and persistent thoughts, impulses, or images that are experienced as intrusive and inappropriate and cause anxiety or distress
- thoughts, impulses, or images that are not simply excessive worries about real-life problems
- attempts to ignore or suppress such thoughts, impulses, or images
- awareness that the obsessional thoughts, impulses, or images are a product of his or her own mind

Compulsions are defined by:

- repetitive behaviors (hand washing, ordering, checking) or mental acts (praying, counting, repeating words silently) that the person feels driven to perform in response to an obsession, or according to rules that must be applied rigidly
- behaviors or mental acts aimed at preventing or reducing distress or preventing some dreaded event or situation

If you recognize that you have obsessive-compulsive disorder, seek help. Far too many people live their lives hiding these problems and not getting the treatment that can make such a difference in the quality of their life.

What is panic disorder?

Panic disorder, a more extreme form of anxiety, is marked by intense episodes of anxiety, usually accompanied by a fear of impending death. These episodes are called *panic attacks.* Once a person has a panic attack, he or she often has an overwhelming fear of future attacks and avoids many situations as a strategy to prevent them. Panic attacks are a painful and debilitating illness.

> *Ten days after I had my son, I had my first experience of thinking I was going to die. I was giving him a bath. Suddenly my heart started pounding. I became dizzy and short of breath. I was so afraid I would pass out that I got on the floor and crawled with the baby into the bedroom. I called my husband, and he came home.*
>
> *I thought I was having a heart attack, so we went to the emergency room. I was crying and worrying about not seeing my baby grow up. They ran tests and told me it was anxiety. I didn't believe them. I called my own doctor, and he ran some more tests.*
>
> *When I kept having panic attacks,, I started reading about panic. I went to a therapist who helped me manage my symptoms and my thinking. Now I can head panic off most of the time. I still can remember how scared I was. It is hard to believe that it is anxiety and that I am not dying.*

Twenty-eight-year-old Melissa's description of her *panic attack* is very typical of first-time sufferers. Panic attacks are terrifying and are often mistaken for heart attacks or strokes.

Many people have experienced moments of panic in frightening situations such as accidents, but this is a normal response to a situation outside the range of typical human experience. Panic attacks occur even when the situation does not warrant the body responding in such a way.

Panic Attack Criteria

A panic attack is a discrete period of intense fear or discomfort, in which four or more of the following symptoms develop abruptly and reach a peak within ten minutes:

- palpitations (sensation of pounding heart) or faster heart rate
- sweating
- trembling or shaking
- shortness of breath or smothering sensations
- feeling of choking
- chest pain or discomfort
- nausea or abdominal distress
- feeling dizzy, unsteady, light-headed or faint
- a sensation that things are not real (derealization or a sensation of being detached from oneself)
- fear of losing control or going crazy
- fear of dying
- numbness or tingling in the hands or feet
- feeling chilled or having hot flashes

Often the panic attack is associated with a certain place or event. Avoiding situations that may precipitate a panic attack becomes a way of life that usually becomes more and more restrictive. For example, let's say you have a panic attack as you're driving and approach a red light. You begin to experience shortness of breath. Heart-pounding thoughts like, "What if I pass out?" or "What if I crash?" begin to race through your head. In the future, you will probably associate red lights with a panicky feeling. Soon you will begin to avoid stoplights and will take long detours to reach your destination. These avoidance strategies create major problems in the life of a person with panic disorder. All types of situations are seen as dangers to be avoided. Soon the world becomes smaller and smaller. Eventually, the person may not be able to leave the house, go into a public building, drive a car, or be around strangers. This creates a fear called agoraphobia, which often accompanies panic episodes.

Agoraphobia, translated literally is "fear of the marketplace." The condition has been known since the time of the ancient Greeks. Individuals with agoraphobia are usually terrified of leaving their homes alone. They may fear such things as being in public or among crowds, standing in a line, being on a bridge, or traveling in a bus or car. This avoidance of public places severely restricts the lives of those with this disorder. Often they will become depressed because they are so isolated. This sense of being alone in a terrifying world and unable to seek help is a very frightening experience.

Sandy, a twenty-two-year-old new mother, illustrates the emotional devastation that can result from agoraphobia and panic attacks:

> *I was driving to the grocery store with the baby for the first time. Six blocks from home, my heart started pounding. I was sweating. I thought I was going to faint. I went back home. I didn't tell anyone because I didn't want to worry them. Somehow I felt ashamed because I*

thought I should be able to do something as simple as go to the store.

I thought maybe I was still tired from the delivery or was anemic. But it kept happening when I drove, so I made up excuses not to drive. I refused to go out of the house for four months.

Finally my husband got impatient with me and made me go out. We got a sitter and went out. I had such a horrible time because I was so scared and wouldn't let go of his hand.

He made me go to see a counselor, and I found out I was having panic attacks. I never knew other people had the same thing. I was able to control my anxiety by breathing. I didn't need medication. I worry that I will have it again if I have another baby.

Sandy's story is tragic. Not only did she have a frightening experience, but she thought she was the only one affected with the problem. Her story also illustrates how people with anxiety may try to hide what is happening to them because they feel a sense of shame. Anxiety becomes a prison that keeps getting smaller and smaller.

If you or someone you know suffers from any of the anxiety disorders described in this chapter, seek help immediately. Like depression, anxiety is very responsive to treatment. Many people have these problems, so you are not alone.

Strategies for managing anxiety

In addition to medication and therapy, there are some strategies you can use to help lessen and eventually prevent anxiety episodes. The most common technique is *relaxation breathing*. Most of us breathe with only part of our lung capacity. We usually do not use our abdominal muscles. By deep breathing and using your abdominal muscles, you can tell your body and mind, "All is well, and you can relax."

Follow the instructions below to learn this breathing relaxation technique:

Relaxation Breathing Instruction

- Sit or lie comfortably. Close your eyes or gaze at a fixed spot in the room.
- Begin to focus on your breathing putting all other thoughts out of your mind. The only thing you have to do now is to practice relaxation breathing.
- Begin to pace your breathing by counting: "in-2-3-4, out-2-3-4." You can also pace your breathing with positive sayings like (breathing in) "I-am-more-relaxed-and-calm, I-am-more-relaxed-and-calm" (breathing out).
- Gradually take deeper and deeper breaths, consciously raising your abdomen when you breathe in and lowering your abdomen when you breathe out.
- Continue comfortably breathing for at least ten minutes.

Like any skill, this will take some practice. Do this for at least five minutes two or three times daily. Gradually, you will develop an automatic response to beginning this kind of breathing. You can use this breathing to help diminish your anxiety or even to prevent anxiety in situations that might create tenseness for you. This kind of behavior training is commonly used to help people lessen their reliance on medication.

A similar technique often used in conjunction with relaxation breathing is *muscle relaxation*. This is usually a guided relaxation exercise; it can be on tape or read to you by someone. You can tape record the steps yourself, but you may find it more helpful to have someone read the steps to you slowly, allowing you to concentrate on the breathing and relaxation:

Progressive Relaxation Routine

- Sit or lie comfortably. Close your eyes or gaze at a spot in the room. Gradually focus your mind on your breathing.
- Begin to take deeper breaths, raising your abdomen as you breathe in and lower your abdomen as your breathe out.
- Feel your body relax and become warmer and heavier as you continue the deep breathing.
- Curl your toes under on both feet and hold for a count of 1-2-3-4. Relax your toes and take two deep breaths.
- Curl your toes under again for a count of 1-2-3-4-5-6. Relax and breathe deeply, being sure your abdomen rises as you breathe in and falls as you breathe out.
- Now tighten your calf muscles for a count of 1-2-3-4.
- Relax and take two deep breaths.
- Tighten your calf muscles again for a count of 1-2-3-4-5-6.
- Let go and breathe deeply, making sure your abdomen rises as you breathe in and falls as you breathe out. Continue this tightening-release-tightening longer-release pattern with your thigh muscles squeezed together, then your buttock muscles, then your abdomen.
- Then continue pattern by clenching your hands into fists, then bending your forearms to the biceps, then shrugging your shoulders.

- Finish with the facial muscles by squinting your eyes, then opening your mouth as far as possible.
- Be sure to deep breathe after tensing each muscle group and count in a gentle rhythmic manner, tensing with the second tensing longer than the first.
- Notice how much more relaxed you feel. You feel calm, relaxed, and peaceful. Tell yourself you have just given your body and mind a treat. It feels good.
- Open your eyes when ready.

You can tape someone reading this for you, or you can tape it yourself, being sure to pace the reading so that you don't rush through it. As with relaxation breathing, consistent practice on a daily basis will develop your capacity to relax in stressful situations.

4

The Spectrum of Postpartum Depression

After my second baby was born, I felt like I never enjoyed her. I resented her crying and felt like I couldn't get enough sleep. I had the blues after my first child, but after about three weeks, I got to feeling better.

After two months of feeling sorry for my baby girl for having such a terrible mother and even wishing I were dead, I told my husband. He had noticed I was irritable and had lost a lot of weight. I hadn't realized I was getting so thin.

I called my OB physician, who sent me to a therapist. I was started on medication and went to therapy for a few months. I didn't realize what I was feeling was so serious.

Carla, a twenty-six-year-old mother of two, describes a very common experience among women with postpartum depression. *Depression* is a mood disorder that affects how we think and feel. The primary pattern of thinking is negative. Thoughts like "I can't stand this any more" or "I will never feel better" are examples of thinking related to depression. The predominant feelings experienced are hopelessness, sadness, and dejection. Some people describe depression as always being in a gray fog with no bright spots. Others describe it as a "numb" sensation. Depression can affect us physically by altering our sleep, appetite, physical movements, and immune system. Physical aches, such as headaches, may be related to depression. Constant fatigue may also be related to depression. New mothers are always fatigued! Depression can affect our ability to solve problems and think rationally. People who are depressed describe their problems focusing or an inability to expend the effort to concentrate.

Postpartum depression, like other kinds of depression, can range from mild to severe states. Here I focus primarily on *major depression*, the most common kind of depression that occurs in the postpartum period. The symptoms must have been present for two weeks to meet the criteria for diagnosis. (Symptons listed in this chapter are from the *Diagnostic and Statistical Manual.*)

Are you having any of these symptoms?

- Do you have thoughts of hurting yourself or the baby?
- Are you planning to kill yourself and the baby?
- Are you hearing voices (Hallucinations)?
- Are you having ideas that you know are not grounded in reality (Delusions)?
- Have you gone more than seventy-two hours without sleep?

If so, consult your physician or mental health professional immediately.

Symptoms of Major Depression

- depressed mood most of the day, nearly every day
- markedly diminished interest or pleasure in all or almost all activities most of the day, nearly every day
- significant weight loss when not dieting, or weight gain, or decrease or increase in appetite nearly every day

- insomnia (inability to sleep) or hypersomnia (sleeping too much) nearly every day
- agitation or slowed movements nearly every day
- fatigue or loss of energy nearly every day
- feelings of worthlessness or excessive or inappropriate guilt
- diminished ability to think and concentrate, or indecisiveness, nearly every day
- recurrent thoughts of death or suicide

There are other kinds of depression. *Dysthymia* is a long-lasting but mild depression. Sometimes dysthymia becomes worse and increases in severity so that an episode of major depression occurs. Dysthymia is commonly found in people who have suffered trauma such as physical or sexual abuse or neglect in their childhood. Dysthymia can develop during adulthood if stress or trauma such as an abusive relationship continues for a period of time. Many people live with dysthymia for long periods of time, thinking they are just tired or stressed.

Symptoms of Dysthymic Disorder

- depressed mood for most of the day, for more days than not, for at least two years
- presence of two or more of the following:
  - poor appetite or overeating
  - insomnia or hypersomnia
  - low energy or fatigue
  - low self-esteem
  - poor concentration or difficulty making decisions
  - feelings of hopelessness
  - symptoms are not due to substance abuse or a medical condition

– symptoms cause significant distress or impairment in social, occupational, or other important functions

Another kind of depression,*bipolar disorder,* is more commonly known as, *manic-depressive disorder.* This kind of depression is characterized by mood swings. At one point, a person with this illness may be very "high," euphoric, even out of touch with reality. This is *mania,* or a *manic episode.* Then the person may experience a slump and become depressed. These cycles may be erratic or regular. There is a strong genetic component to this disorder. It is important for women with severe symptoms to understand this illness because a first diagnosis of bipolar disorder is often made during the postpartum period.

There are several categories of bipolar disorders. The criteria for diagnosing a manic episode are described below.

Criteria for Manic Episode Diagnosis

- a distinct period of abnormally and persistently elevated, expansive, or irritable moods
- three or more of the following symptoms are present during an episode:
  – inflated self-esteem or grandiosity
  – decreased need of sleep
  – more talkative than usual or pressure to keep talking
  – flight of ideas (unable to stay on one topic, racing thoughts)
  – distractibility, or inability to focus on a task or idea
  – excessive movements, inability to be quiet, and/or agitation

- excessive involvement in pleasurable activities that have a high potential for self-harm, such as buying sprees, business risks, sexual activity, or physical risks
- the symptoms are severe enough to cause marked impairment in occupational or social functions, or to require hospitalization of self or others, or there are psychotic features
- the symptoms are not due to the effects of a drug or medication or a general medical condition such as hyperthyroidism

Diagnosing mood disorders is sometimes very difficult because a person may show symptoms of more than one kind of depression.

How postpartum depression differs from other depressive disorders.

The criteria used to diagnose postpartum depression are not specific to postpartum states. In addition to the previously listed symptoms, the unique aspects of depression in women who have had a baby usually include an extreme fear of some harm coming to the baby and fear or feelings of guilt about being a "bad" mother. These thoughts are the hallmark of postpartum depression and distinguish it from other kinds of depression. Carla describes her experience:

When I look back at what I was thinking when I was so depressed, it really scares me. The emotional pain was so great that I lost my perspective about me. I never thought I would ever want to kill myself, yet at the time it seemed like such a logical solution to the pain. I still feel guilty that I could ever think about hurting my baby. I still have to work at the idea that those thoughts were depression, not the real me.

One of the most troublesome facets of any kind of depression is that it affects our perception of ourselves and the world. We don't think that something is happening "to" us. Rather, we think we "are" that something. Paula did not realize she was depressed. She could not objectively observe her negative thoughts and feelings. When you have a cold, you realize there is a change in your health. You say, "I have a cold," rather than "I am a cold." But with depression, you think, "I am depressed," rather than "I have a depression." This perception, as well as the shame and embarrassment associated with mental illness, keeps women from talking about their internal experiences.

The most severe form of depression brings suicidal and homicidal thoughts. When a woman feels so bad that she thinks she cannot take it anymore and that there is no hope for change, the future looks very bleak. When the situation seems hopeless, some women begin to think that they and their baby would be better off dead. This reaction seems like an extreme one to those who are not suffering the pain and agony of depression. Unfortunately, for anyone who is very depressed, death may seem like a logical alternative.

The good news is that major depression is a very treatable illness. With prompt treatment, the response is usually quick. In fact, one recent study shows that women with postpartum depression respond faster and require less medication than those with other kinds of depression.

Why does depression occur?

If you are like most people, you probably find depression difficult to understand. Even more confusing is why the time after having a baby may be so hard for you. You are not alone. Psychiatric clinicians and researchers are not entirely certain why the postpartum period is a time of high risk for an adult woman to become depressed.

In general, after adolescence, women are twice as likely to experience depression than men. Many factors—sociological, psychological, and physiological—contribute to this alarming statistic. Violence such as rape or sexual abuse may be a major cause of depression. Women are much more likely to experience such violence than men. Psychological and sociological stress interacts with biology in a way that we do not yet fully understand. You must think of yourself as a whole person, not as a body with a separate mind. As Dana C. Jack states in *Silencing the Self: Women and Depression*:

> *…depression is a complex and multifaceted illness. By current consensus, major depression results from an interaction of biological and psychosocial factors; no single cause can be isolated. Given that psychological stresses translate into biochemical changes within the brain, the distinction between physical and social factors may be artificial….*

As I mentioned earlier, one of the major predictors for postpartum mood disorders is the prior experience of mood changes during the menstrual cycle. Most research indicates that there may be a hormonal component to some female mood disorders, but our current understanding of the complex endocrine system is incomplete. Otherwise, all women (who have similar hormones) would experience mood disorders. Statistically, the time after delivery is an adult woman's greatest period of risk for a psychiatric disorder, and it is also the time of greatest fluctuation in hormone levels. Abrupt hormonal changes may be a major factor in mood changes after delivery.

During pregnancy, hormone levels are high because the placenta produces hormones. Your female hormones—*estrogens* and *progesterones*—are at a very high level. Your level of male hormones, or *androgens*, is also high because they rise in proportion to the levels of your female hormones. The thyroid gland also increases production during pregnancy. At delivery, removal of the placenta and fetus causes the female and male hormone levels to drop drastically. At the same time, *prolactin*, a hormone that promotes milk production, increases. The prolactin level remains high for about two weeks after delivery, regardless of whether you are breast-feeding. Studies that have evaluated the use of hormones to treat mood changes during the postpartum period are inconclusive as yet. The complex relationship of your endocrine system to moods and thoughts is not yet very well understood.

As we've established, women who have had a previous major depression or anxiety episode are also at greater risk of postpartum depression. Why? The "kindling theory" suggests that once a person has a mood disorder, he or she is more susceptible to further episodes of mood disorders. This may be due to a vulnerability to altered levels of chemicals, called *neurotransmitters*, in the brain. This, too, is not well understood, and research is ongoing. Carla had an earlier episode of depression in college, although she did not realize its significance at the time:

> *I remember a time in college when I was depressed for about six months. I barely kept up in class, lost weight, slept a lot, and even lost a lot of my friends. I thought I was just stressed, but now I realize I was depressed. I thought my thoughts of wanting to be dead were just because I was so tired all the time.*

Carla's experience is not at all uncommon. Many people can have a mood disorder and not realize what is happening to them.

There also appear to be genetic influences on major depression. As yet, the role of genetics and heredity is not well understood. However, a positive family history does not automatically mean that you will not develop depression.

The postpartum period is filled with major stress and fatigue that affects your adjustment. Whether one or the other causes depression remains unclear. It may very well be an interaction among all the variables.

Stressful events in life such as moving, job loss, the death of a loved one, or financial reversal, appear to play a significant role in precipitating a depressive episode. Stress may play a role in altering the chemicals in the brain that influence our moods. This phenomenon is not unique to childbearing, but the increased vulnerability and dependency inherent in having a child may place women more at risk.

The quality of a woman's relationship with her partner or spouse is another very important variable in determining one's vulnerability to depression. According to several studies, lower levels of marital satisfaction and lack of support are key factors in postpartum depression. If your relationship with your significant other is strained, the new baby in your life may feel like more of a burden or may make you feel more "trapped."

Psychologically, the postpartum period forces you to assume a new identity and role. Sometimes the baby seems larger than life. You may often feel overwhelmed by the monumental change that has just occurred. Part of this new identity involves adjusting to the changes in your body. All women (in fact, all parents) will have some mixed feelings about this new intrusion and change in their lives. *Ambivalence* will occur even if the pregnancy was very much planned and wanted. Any change involves loss, and loss includes some conflicting emotions, even when the change is a positive one. The losses include the sense of oneself and the loss of the "couple," for now there are three instead of two. Freedom of choice and one's sense of control may be stolen by this new, totally dependent little person. Sometimes the baby's arrival even signifies loss. Maybe now you will never finish school, get that degree, move to another part of the country, and so on.

The mother's psychological makeup may have some bearing on her tendency to become depressed. Again, this is not unique to the postpartum period. Women who have negative, critical, or blaming thoughts about themselves are more likely to become depressed. Women who need to feel in control or to maintain perfectionism are also at risk of depression. Because the postpartum time is particularly stressful, the new mother facing greater responsibilities and lacking typical coping mechanisms will be at risk for postpartum depression.

So how do you put all the various factors together that may contribute to postpartum depression? In his work, *Psychological*

Aspects of Women's Reproductive Health, Dr. Michael O'Hara summarizes these factors:

> *...a "composite sketch" of the woman who is most likely to be at risk can be developed. The vulnerable pregnant woman is one who has had a past episode of depression (or other serious psychiatric disorders). During pregnancy or after delivery, she may experience some significant negative life events such as loss of housing or loss of employment for herself or her partner. She may be in an unsatisfying relationship with her partner, or she may have no partner to provide support and assistance to her. Finally, during the early postpartum period she may experience the blues, which may persist longer than usual. All of these features will increase the woman's risk for a postpartum depression.*

How does maternal depression affect the baby?

The mother-infant connection is vital to the mental and physical health of the baby. Anything that interferes with the critical process of bonding will have a detrimental effect. Depression only makes the new mother less able to respond to the needs of the infant.

However, we must not underestimate the hardiness of the baby. Dr. Martin Maldonado, child psychiatrist and professor at the Karl Menninger School of Psychiatry, says, "Babies are quite resilient and don't give up easily. They have a big repertoire of behaviors to make parents respond." He describes several signs that a baby might be affected by a mother's mood changes: mild delays in speech, too placid or content, too irritable, short attention span, feeding difficulties, sleep problems, and a depressed look on the baby's face. "Problems have multiple causes, and it is not helpful to find blame," he cautions parents. Maldonado also proposes that if problems exist for the baby, then attention should be paid to the whole family, especially the mother.

A new mother who is depressed or anxious will not be as sensitive to her baby as a mother who is not depressed. A mother who is depressed will show less affection toward her baby, will be less attentive and responsive to the baby's cues, and may even demonstrate hostile actions toward the baby. *Attunement,* the mother's "knowing" her baby and his or her needs, is crucial in mother-infant relationships. A mother who is depressed or anxious will not be as attuned to the baby. In addition, babies pick up cues from their parents and imitate them. A woman who is depressed will show more negative cues like frowning or not smiling or other unhappy expressions. As a result, the baby will learn a more restricted range of emotional expressions.

It is difficult to predict the impact of the mother's illness on the baby due to the multitude of contributing factors: the severity of her illness, its duration, the number of other people involved with the baby, and the baby's temperament. In general, mothers who are depressed during their baby's first year of life may have a negative impact on their child's development. Various studies measuring that effect have found that the more depressed the mother, the greater the delay in the infant's development. The first year is a particularly critical time for cognitive development. If development is delayed, the effects may still be evident years later. In the words of Cheryl Beck, Ph.D., a nurse and researcher:

It is imperative that greater attention be paid to de-pressed mother and infant. Rapidly developing infants experience the world through those who care for them. Most times, the mother constitutes the primary social environment in the months after birth. Early identification and resolution of postpartum depression will help to alleviate disturbances in mother-infant interactions and enhance the development of warm, sensitive relationships.

What about the rest of the family?

Postpartum depression involves more people than just you and your baby. Other family members will also be confused and concerned. After all, they think, most women don't feel this way. Relatives may downplay the problem or blame the mother, which can delay treatment. Yet family members are in a unique position to recognize the problem and to help make the new mother aware of her depression. Their lack of information about postpartum mood disorders, however, may prevent them from realizing that this is a real problem that requires treatment to avoid the sometimes tragic consequences.

Sam, a thirty-one-year-old father of two, speaks to the double tragedy of postpartum mood disorders.

My wife had some problems with crying and thinking she was a bad mother after the birth of our first baby. After our second was born, it was worse. She didn't want to be left alone with the baby and didn't even want to touch it. I had to work, and it was a terrible time for us.

When the baby was one month old, I got a call from my neighbor. My wife had left the kids with her and said she couldn't stand to hurt her kids any more and left. I didn't see her for about four years, and I didn't know if

*she was dead or alive. We divorced, and she has very lit-
tle contact with the children. I found out some information about postpartum depression. I wish I would have
known. Maybe my kids would have had their mother.*

This is a tragic example of how the lack of information and
treatment can have devastating results for a family.

What is the treatment for postpartum depression?

Once a diagnosis of postpartum depression is made, treatment usually consists of medication, therapy, or a combination of
the two. There is controversy about which approach is most effective, but a general consensus exists that both together are
more effective than either one alone.

If you have never been in therapy or talked with a mental
health professional, you will probably feel anxious. The process
usually includes an evaluation by a clinician, which involves asking questions about your past medical and psychiatric history,
your family history, and the severity and range of your symptoms. The clinician will then determine the diagnosis.

Mood management strategies

If you are having problems like those described in this chapter, the most important step to take is to obtain professional help.
In addition, you can help yourself by reading and becoming
more knowledgeable about depression.

Minimizing stress in your life will help you get better. If you
can take an extended leave of absence from work or ask someone to care for your other children for a period of time, you can

make your recovery a priority. It is sometimes difficult for mothers to realize that they can help their children and family the most by taking care of themselves first.

Another strategy is to ask for help. Sometimes the people around us do not realize we are having trouble. Be clear and direct about what you would like people to do. Allow others to take responsibility. Give yourself permission to heal. Recovering from a major depressive episode will take longer than you think. And, it requires an effort on your part to change. This effort requires energy and concentration that you will not have if you expend your time and energy on things other people can do for you, such as housecleaning and cooking.

Eating a healthful diet, avoiding alcohol and caffeine, and getting some physical exercise daily will also help you get better. Now is a good time to incorporate some physically healthy habits into your routine that will also help you manage your moods.

Postpartum psychotic depression

Confusion, paranoia, agitation, and hallucinations are all symptoms of a severe postpartum illness called *postpartum psychotic depression*. Psychosis is characterized by delusions (false ideas), such as the thought that someone has bugged your phone, and hallucinations, which involve seeing, hearing, smelling, or feeling things that are not really there, such as seeing someone in the wallpaper. In addition, disorganized speech and disorganized behavior are present. Many people think that psychotic behavior indicates the presence of schizophrenia—a disorder in the brain causing severe, long-term mental illness. But there are many causes of psychosis, and schizophrenia is just one. By far, the vast majority of women who have postpartum psychosis are not affected by schizophrenia.

Postpartum psychosis is a perplexing illness for both the mother and those treating her. Whether it is one illness or a combination of similar illnesses is not clear. In general, the disorder is usually viewed as a severe form of depression called *bipolar depression* and is unrelated to other psychotic disorders. As such, postpartum psychotic depression differs from major depression in its time of onset and its symptoms. This disorder usually begins postpartum within three to ten days. It is characterized by agitation, insomnia, hallucinations, and delusions. The disorder must have appeared no more than four weeks after delivery to be considered postpartum. The following story by June, an R.N. in an obstetrician's office, describes a typical woman with postpartum *psychotic* depression.

> *We got a call from the husband of one of our patients, who came home from a business trip and found his wife putting their four-day-old baby in the trash in the garage. The baby was filthy and hungry and had been neglected. His wife was claiming the baby had been taken by Satan. She was dirty, confused, had a raging breast infection, and was psychotic.*
>
> *We hospitalized her. She responded very quickly and was home within a week. She was mortified at what she had done. We really had to work with her to let her know that she was ill and that we knew she loved her baby. The sad thing is, her sister had had a similar problem, but she never told our patient, so she did not know about this illness.*

Symptoms of Brief Psychotic Disorder

- presence of one or more of the following symptoms:
  - delusions
  - hallucinations
  - disorganized speech
  - grossly disorganized behavior
- the symptoms last at least one day and less than one month

One difficulty in detecting a psychotic state is that there may be periods when a woman is more in touch with reality. In addition, sometimes women do not reveal that they are having strange thoughts and experiences. Immediately after childbirth is the time of highest risk for a woman to become psychotic. It is not clear why this happens to about 1 of every 1,000 women after delivery.

The onset of psychosis is usually preceded by a time of marked agitation, restlessness, and insomnia. Sonya, a first-time mother at age thirty, describes her experience with postpartum psychosis:

> *I don't remember much, except that I was agitated, both physically and mentally. My thoughts were going fast, and I could not focus on any one thing at all. I even remember some thoughts I had about the baby being evil, and I thought I saw yellow vapor come from his mouth. I did not know anything was wrong, and no one else realized it for several days after I was home. I look back now and am terrified about what could have happened.*

As with Sonya, it may be impossible to detect postpartum psychosis immediately. But a woman who is becoming psychotic will begin to behave in a noticeably bizarre manner. Both the baby and the mother are at risk during this time because the new mother's judgment is quite impaired. This illness should be considered an emergency, and urgent measures must be taken to bring the situation under control.

If the psychosis goes unrecognized and untreated, the mother may harm her baby or herself. This tragedy can often be avoided by obstetric and pediatric clinicians who know how to recognize the signs of postpartum psychosis. Since postpartum psychosis usually develops soon after delivery, signs may be present as early as the first day. Extreme restlessness and agitation after delivery and an inability to sleep the first night are early clues. The mother may complain of being confused or disoriented, or of feeling "strange."

What is the treatment for postpartum psychotic depression?

Postpartum psychosis presents a crisis for the family. The husband and other relatives may not understand what is happening if this is the woman's first episode of psychiatric difficulties. Most families think that the illness indicates the mother will never be able to care for her baby, which is not true. Sonya's husband, Guy, describes his fears:

> *I thought I had lost my wife and would have to raise the baby myself. I had never heard of postpartum psychosis, so I thought she would always be hallucinating and delusional. I was so relieved when she became her old self again. But I will never forget how scared I was that Sonya would never get any better.*

Most women respond rapidly to treatment and can quickly resume care of the child. Most women also will never have another episode of psychosis unless they have another baby. Then their risk of a second episode of postpartum psychosis is significant.

Postpartum psychosis must be treated promptly. To protect both the woman and her baby, initial treatment usually includes hospitalization. Until the mother becomes stabilized, the baby must be cared for by someone else. Some hospitals allow the baby to room with the mother when another person is there to care for the baby. Most hospitals in the United States, however, do not allow such arrangements.

The aftereffects of postpartum psychosis may last much longer than the psychosis itself. Sonya states,

> *It took me a long time to get over the shame of having postpartum psychosis. I kept watching myself for signs that I might not be over it. I never want to go through that again, but I want to have another baby. We haven't decided what to do.*

What about future postpartum risks after a psychotic depression episode?

A woman with postpartum psychosis is at risk of future postpartum psychotic episodes, and all of her health care providers should be so informed. Some experts estimate this risk to be as high as 40 to 60 percent. One study shows the risk to be 100 percent if the previous episode occurred within the past twenty-four months.

There have been some attempts to prevent recurrences in women known to be at risk. But these preventive measures have been based on small samples, so further research is needed. The mood stabilizer lithium has been given to women after delivery to prevent postpartum psychosis. Researcher Dr. Deborah Sichel has also reported on the use of estrogen after delivery to prevent the development of mood disorders. She hypothesizes that the change in estrogen levels after delivery may cause an "estrogen withdrawal state" that causes the extreme mood swings. Because Sichel's study involved a small number of women, however, caution is advised in using estrogen after delivery until more research is completed.

5

Navigating the Mental Health System

> *I knew I needed help. I had read several books about depression when I was trying to figure out why I was crying all the time, couldn't get things done, and didn't want to be around my baby. My sister had some depression once, and she went to a therapist. I had no idea how to find someone that I could trust. I called my doctor, and he gave me some names. I was really scared because I didn't know what to expect. I was also afraid of the stigma of "mental illness."*
>
> Amanda, new mother

Amanda's lack of knowledge about mental health professionals and her apprehension about getting help for her depression are common experiences among women suffering postpartum depression or anxiety. Seeking treatment can be unsettling when you are not familiar with psychiatric professionals and your options for care. This chapter is your guide to psychiatric treatment, from the different psychiatric professionals to the variety of treatment options. Unfortunately, there is little specific treatment unique to postpartum disorders. Much of the information included here is adapted from standard treatment protocols for depression and anxiety.

The psychiatric treatment you receive depends on the type of health care professional you consult. This is true for psychiatric disorders in general, not just postpartum disorders. When an obstetrician, family practice physician, or nurse-practitioner treats a person with a mood disorder, medication is commonly prescribed. Most medications for psychiatric disorders are initially prescribed by nonpsychiatric health care professionals. For some people, this treatment may be adequate. If you need further treatment, you will be referred to a mental health professional who can offer therapy in addition to, or instead of, medication.

There are advantages to combining therapy and medication in the treatment of depression or anxiety. Therapy develops skills that will help abate the mood disorder, and it also teaches you to recognize the risk factors and indicators of future mood disorders. Also, medication may help you be more responsive to therapy, although some people respond to individual or group therapy and other nonmedication treatments so well that they may not need medication. A mental health professional is more likely to be knowledgeable about the wide range of treatment options. The information about treatment in this chapter assumes that you are consulting with a mental health professional or are considering doing so.

What can I expect?

Whether you are referred to a specific mental health professional or you are calling an agency on your own, you can expect to encounter a similar process. You will be asked to come in to register, which is similar to the kind of paperwork required by obstetricians and other health care providers. You will meet with an intake worker, who may be the mental health professional with whom you will work. During this intake or consultation session, you will be asked a series of in-depth questions. The intake session will usually last forty-five to sixty minutes so that the mental health professional will have enough time to understand not only your current symptoms but also how those symptoms compare with how you felt at earlier times in your life. Another reason for in-depth questioning is that psychiatric symptoms can have multiple causes, so it is important for the professional to understand as much about you as possible.

During a counseling session, common intake interview questions include:

- Why are you seeking treatment?
- What are your current symptoms?
- What is your past psychiatric history?
- What is your past medical history?
  Medications you are taking, drug allergies, and illnesses or surgeries. Use of caffeine, alcohol, nicotine, and other substances.
- What is your family history?
  The clinician may prepare a *genogram,* a type of family tree. Questions will focus on past and present relationships in your family, family use of alcohol and drugs, any history of drug abuse, and psychiatric and medical illnesses.
- What is your current life like? Your work, social activities, interests, support systems, relationships, and any stresses in your life?

- Questions will also focus on your memory and thought patterns.

After obtaining a description of your history and current complaints, the mental health clinician will likely conclude with an assessment and a diagnosis as well as options for treatment. To determine the diagnosis, the mental health professional will consult the *Diagnostic and Statistical Manual,* used by mental health professionals to ensure consistency in diagnosis. In addition, most insurance companies require the use of this manual for payment.

In addition, a thorough medical history will be taken as well because it is standard practice in psychiatric treatment to rule out any physical causes. Many medical disorders, including hypothyroidism, hyperthyroidism, and anemia, can cause symptoms of depression and anxiety. Lab tests may also be recommended. If you do not agree with or are concerned about either the diagnosis or the recommendations, then you should seek a second opinion.

At this point, you can also ask questions and participate in formulating the treatment plan. The more information you have, the better your decision will be. Keep in mind that the decision about any recommended psychiatric treatment is yours to make.

What are the types of mental health professionals?

There are four main groups of mental health professionals from whom you might commonly seek treatment for a postpartum disorder: advanced practice nurses, social workers, psychologists, and psychiatrists.

Advanced practice nurse: A registered nurse with a master's degree in psychiatric nursing. Graduate preparation includes a clinical practicum in a mental health setting. These nurses may also be called *clinical nurse specialists* or *advanced registered nurse practitioners.* In some states they prescribe medications for common psychiatric disorders. These nurses are licensed R.N.s who usually have a certification if their state recognizes advanced practice nurses. There is a voluntary national certification program for child and adolescent advanced practice nurses and for adult advanced practice nurses. Some nurses may also have a Ph.D.

Social worker: A master's level graduate who has completed a clinical practicum as part of a graduate program. Since some social workers are not clinically trained but instead provide other kinds of services, be sure to ask about their clinical preparation. Other titles in this category include *licensed specialist clinical social worker* (LSCSW) and *clinical social worker* (CSW). There is a voluntary national certification for social workers. Some social workers may also have a Ph.D.

Psychologist: A doctoral level graduate who has completed a graduate academic program with a required clinical component. Some psychologists are not clinical psychologists. (Social psychologists, for example, are not qualified to do therapy.) Other titles these professionals use may be *clinical psychologist* (Ph.D.) or *doctorate in psychology* (PsyD). Some states recognize master's degree programs in psychology, whose graduates are also known as psychologists. Be sure either the master's or Ph.D. level clinician you consult has clinical graduate program experience. There is national certification for psychologists.

Psychiatrist: A physician who has completed medical school and has an M.D. or D.O. degree. The graduate program following medical school is called a *residency* and usually takes four years or longer. The residency training may involve children, adults, or both. Be sure the psychiatrist you consult has completed a residency in psychiatry. Other specialties have residency programs also. Psychiatrists may be nationally certified.

All four of the primary types of mental health professionals are licensed by the state in which they live or practice, so the titles and requirements among states vary. Each professional group has a national certifying body that assures minimum standards. Certification is not required to practice, however.

Other professionals also may offer therapy; these include marriage/family therapists, ministers, and licensed counselors. Their qualifications may vary. In some states psychotherapy is unregulated, so anyone may call himself a *psychotherapist*. Understanding the credentials of mental health professionals can help you make a good decision about the right therapist for you.

What kind of mental health professional should I see?

Deciding on a mental health professional can be difficult. Unlike the medical field, where roles are more distinct, many kinds of mental health clinicians do much the same kind of work. According to *Consumer Reports*, 4,000 readers responded to a survey on satisfaction with mental health providers. The results indicate, "people were just as satisfied and reported similar progress whether they saw a social worker, psychologist, or a psychiatrist."

Your choice of therapists may depend on the availability of clinicians in your area. Another factor is the cost of treatment. If you are paying for treatment yourself, master's level clinicians like advanced practice nurses and social workers may be less expensive. If you have insurance, your policy may dictate which kind of professional you can see. If you are participating in an HMO or PPO, there may be restrictions on whom you can see. Two types of providers may prescribe medication: advanced practice nurses and psychiatrists. It is not uncommon for a person to see both a clinician who cannot prescribe (such as a social worker) for therapy and a clinician who prescribes medication.

Just as important as the kind of therapist is the kind of therapy offered. To further add to the confusion in this field, there are several different kinds of theoretical approaches that may be used by the four primary mental health providers. In fact, most clinicians use a combination of approaches, describing themselves as eclectic.

What should I look for in a therapist?

When consulting a therapist, you are like any other consumer in search of and paying for a service. You should ask questions, check credentials, and obtain references. You should also interview more than one therapist, because it may not be easy to determine who will best "fit" with you without meeting more than one clinician. Only *you* can determine if you trust and feel comfortable with someone. It is generally not a good idea to go to a therapist you know personally or have contact with on another business or professional basis.

One resource for therapists is Depression after Delivery, a national organization that provides therapy referrals as well as information about postpartum problems. They may have information about someone in your area who is knowledgeable about postpartum disorders.

To help you determine competence, here are some questions to ask the mental health professional:

- Are you licensed to do therapy?
- Are you nationally certified?
- What experience have you had with postpartum mood disorders?
- Have you ever been the subject of a disciplinary action from your state's licensing board?
- What approach or type of therapy do you use?
- What is your plan for emergency coverage?
- What is your fee?

After you have met with a mental health professional, ask yourself these questions:

- Did I feel comfortable talking with him or her? Was I able to be completely open?
- Did I feel that I was being judged or criticized?
- Was the therapist able to help me understand my problem and the plan for treatment, or am I just as confused as before we met?
- Was the focus on me or on the therapist?

You will be better able to answer these questions for yourself after consulting more than one mental health professional.

What kind of therapy is best for postpartum mood disorders?

Two common therapy approaches are most often used for depression and anxiety: *cognitive-behavioral therapy* and *interpersonal therapy*. There are other, less common, approaches that are not discussed here.

Cognitive-behavioral therapy emphasizes the influence of thinking on mood. The relationship of thoughts, feelings, and behaviors on the belief system formed by early childhood experiences will be a primary focus. The basic premise is that depression and anxiety are the result of faulty conclusions formed during childhood. Change can occur by learning new responses and new habits. This approach is sometimes combined with behavioral therapy. The therapist is interactive, provides feedback, and views therapy as a collaborative process. Homework assignments are likely to be given to facilitate change.

Interpersonal therapy is based on a relationship between you and the therapist. The basic premise is that there is a connection between your mood disorder and the current interpersonal relationships in your life. Change occurs by correcting dysfunctional behaviors within a therapeutic relationship. The therapist will be supportive, warm, and understanding, and will focus much of the work on the interaction between the two of you. This kind of therapy may take longer because it takes awhile for trust and a relationship to develop.

How do you decide which approach is best? Unfortunately, no research has shown exactly which ones are best for certain problems. This is very much an individual decision. One factor to consider is your history. If this is the first time you have experienced symptoms of depression or anxiety, and you do not have a history of trauma (like neglect, physical abuse, or sexual abuse), then brief therapy should be your first step. *Relieving the symptoms of your current problem should be the first goal of your treatment.* Initial treatment should not focus on your conflicts with your mother or your ambivalence about having a baby. If the initial treatment does not help you feel better, then you can look at the historical factors that may be affecting you.

Whatever therapy you decide is best, there are some commonalities that make sense for all types of therapy, according to mental health professionals Ivan Miller, Ph.D. and Gabor Keitner, M.D.:

- be clear about the rationale for treatment
- establish a time limit, probably weekly sessions for twelve to twenty-four weeks
- employ a therapist who is active and directive
- focus on current problems
- emphasize changing current behavior
- teach self-monitoring of change
- include homework assignments to facilitate application of what is learned to daily life problems

If anxiety is the primary symptom, many clinicians recommend a cognitive-behavioral approach as the treatment of choice. Because most clinicians use a variety of approaches, be sure to ask which approach the professional is going to use and what the rationale is for that choice.

What about group therapy?

Group therapy involves several patients meeting with one or more therapists in a group setting. The groups may be time-limited or ongoing. They may be structured, meaning there is a set format or agenda for each group session, or the group may be unstructured, which means that the therapist is not directive but will make interpretations about the process of the group. Group therapy is very cost-effective, so managed care companies encourage participation. Group therapy has the advantage of decreasing the sense of isolation that accompanies depression and anxiety. It has the disadvantage of less individual time that is tailored specifically to your own needs.

Group therapy is probably not the best treatment for you initially if you meet the criteria for depression or anxiety disorders. However, it may be a very useful addition to your individual therapy.

Few studies have examined the effects of group treatment on postpartum depression. In one prominent study, however, ten group therapy participants were observed over a ten-week period. The group format involved education, social support, and cognitive-behavioral therapy. When women in the treatment group were compared with women who received no treatment, the depression and self-esteem scores of the participants improved significantly over those of women who did not participate. This small study was an important beginning effort to target treatment for postpartum depression and anxiety.

If you decide to try group therapy, be sure to first ask about the purpose of the group. If the group is designed to educate, support, and promote change toward healthy behaviors, then it may be helpful. But if the purpose is not clearly stated and the time frame is open-ended, you may want to instead choose a type of treatment more immediately helpful to you.

What can I do to help myself?

Exercise has been demonstrated to improve the mood of depressed women. Although studies have not been conducted specifically with postpartum women, we can safely assume that the effects may be the same. Exercise has proved the most effective strategy in changing a "bad" mood into a positive mood compared to other strategies like socializing, distraction, and relaxation techniques. It is not clear whether the exercise must be vigorous or whether a more moderate approach, such as walking, is just as effective. The positive effect of exercise on women's self-esteem even if they are not clinically depressed has been demonstrated in a study of twenty-seven female volunteers who were not clinically depressed. These volunteers participated in an eight-week walking program. In addition to the physical benefits, the women reported an increase in positive self-esteem.

Postpartum women have several reasons to exercise. It provides physical conditioning after pregnancy that will help the body return to its pre-pregnant state. It will help improve the overall health of women with children who are already stressed due to a lack of sleep. Physical activity helps promote sleep. If you are depressed, you may find it harder to make yourself exercise. Having a friend or another mother join you may help motivate you until the exercise routine becomes a habit. A scheduled exercise time that is a pre-planned part of your daily routine will help reinforce your decision to exercise. Although the effects are not dramatic and quick, over time you will notice that you feel better, you have more energy, and your mood is brighter.

In addition to exercise, *diet* can play a significant role in how you feel. Good nutrition is essential for everyone, but it is especially important for people with mood disorders. Excessive amounts of sugar can cause mood changes severe enough to affect your work or concentration. Caffeine can trigger both anxiety and mood changes, so it should be avoided. Alcohol and other drugs can affect mood adversely. In addition, alcohol and other drugs can affect the level of medications present in your body. If used, alcohol should be taken only in moderate amounts, such as one or two drinks per week.

Research has been done on other mood-regulating strategies for both men and women. Besides proper exercise and nutrition, socializing techniques such as talking to others, being with people, and even talking on the phone may help. Distracting techniques such as listening to music, doing housework, and watching TV or reading are used by some people. Cognitive strategies such as giving yourself a "pep talk" or reminding yourself of all the positive aspects of your life might be useful. Passive strategies such as napping or sleeping are helpful to some. Isolating yourself, using alcohol, or blaming yourself for your mood are not helpful strategies.

Once you have found a mental health professional who is helpful and trustworthy, and you have done all you can do to improve your health, the next decision you may face is whether to take medication.

6

Understanding the Use of Medications

Not every woman needs medication. The severity and longevity of your symptoms are the key factors in determining whether to take medication. If you have experienced anxiety or depression over a period of several weeks or months, or if you have had similar symptoms before, untreated or not, taking medication is most likely wise. If your symptoms are so severe that you are having trouble taking care of yourself or the baby, or if you are having suicidal thoughts, medication is strongly recommended. Because your perspective about the illness and its treatment is limited, it is important to listen to the recommendations of your mental health professional. The ultimate decision is yours, though, just as it is about therapy and therapists. If you are not experiencing severe symptoms, and if you have support, it may be feasible to try therapy for a few sessions to see whether it alone will be sufficient. But try to keep an open mind about the possibility of taking medication and using other treatments.

Like many women with postpartum depression, Amanda gained some benefit from psychotherapy, but she also required medication to fully treat her symptoms:

I found a good therapist who helped me feel less de-
pressed, but she recommended that I take an antidepres-
sant in addition to coming to therapy. I didn't want to
take medication—I was afraid I might get sicker. My
therapist gave me some reading material, and I finally
understood how the medication works. I am glad I
agreed to take the medication. It helped me feel so much
better, and I could see myself getting better faster.

As a psychotherapist, I often encounter women in severe distress who say, "Please help me, but I won't take medication." I usually agree to try therapy first, but if they are not feeling significantly better after two or three sessions, I usually recommend medication.

Why are women reluctant to take psychiatric medication?

In my experience, some men and women fear taking antidepressant or anti-anxiety medications. Yet these same people willingly take antibiotics, smoke cigarettes, drink alcohol, or take over-the-counter medications. I believe their fear of psychiatric medication is based on a lack of information or even on misinformation.

Many people with depression or anxiety tell me, "I should be able to fix this myself without having to rely on medication." I then ask them, "If you had diabetes, would you expect to fix it yourself? Or, if you were anemic, would you use will power to change that? Or, if you have an infection, do you expect to counter the bacteria by will power?" I then explain the changes in the brain related to depression or anxiety.

Depression and anxiety result in actual chemical changes in the brain. Or it may be that chemical changes result in the symptoms we call depression and anxiety. There is much we don't know, but most of what we call "mental illness" is an alteration in the neurological or chemical functioning of the brain. Researchers have created depression in laboratory animals by exposing them to prolonged stress, such as noise, temperature changes, and flashing lights. After a period of time, the animals resemble humans who are depressed. They lose interest in playing, they lie in their cages, they won't eat, and they won't greet the attendants as they used to. To cite another example, prisoners of war who were mentally healthy before exposure to trauma or prolonged stress also develop depression and anxiety.

What changes take place in my brain when I am depressed or anxious?

While the brain is still a mystery to us in many ways, we know more today that helps us understand our thoughts and feelings. The brain is composed of over 100 billion nerve cells called *neurons*. These nerve cells transmit information by electrical and chemical changes. Every thought, action, and feeling is the result of these changes throughout the brain. Depression and anxiety are thought to be the results of an excess of, or deficiency in, either the chemical activity or the electrical activity of the brain.

Although there are more than fifty known kinds of neurotransmitters, for the purposes of understanding what happens in depression and anxiety, let's focus on the primary neurotransmitters that affect mood and anxiety: *dopamine, norepinephrine, serotonin*, and transmitters of *GABA* and *glutamate*. These neurotransmitters work together to regulate our thinking, emotions, and behaviors. Dopamine is important in learning, memory, and emotional arousal. You probably have had a frightening experience in your life that you remember vividly. Dopamine is involved in helping you remember the event with such detail. In fact, you might even be able to remember smells, sounds, or other sensory information associated with the experience. Without dopamine, you would not be able to remember events in such intense detail.

Norepinephrine is very similar to adrenaline, the hormone released during stress. Lack of this chemical is related to depression. Too much of this same chemical is related to a state of agitation or mania.

Serotonin seems to play a role in influencing how excited our brain cells get and in helping us fall asleep. Serotonin also plays a major role in regulating mood.

GABA resembles serotonin in that it helps regulate how fast the messages are sent along the nerve cells. Its role is very important because anxiety is considered to be a process of excessive stimulation. A related neurotransmitter is glutamate, which performs the opposite action. Medications that affect the levels of these neurotransmitters will enhance or inhibit brain activity.

In addition to these major neurotransmitters, *endorphins* play a role in regulating mood. These small proteins seem to promote a sense of well-being and happiness. Exercise increases the production and release of endorphins.

The hormones from our endocrine system—both the female estrogen and progesterone and the male hormone testosterone as well as hormones from the thyroid gland—seem to influence the normal functions of nerve cells. The role of the endocrine system in mood regulation is not yet well understood.

The thyroid is an important endocrine gland that may be a factor in postpartum depression. For some reason, massive changes in the body can affect the functions of the entire endocrine system, including the thyroid. In addition, the change in estrogen and progesterone levels may influence mood in some women. The thyroid is often overlooked as a factor in postpartum mood changes. If your health care provider has not ordered a lab test to evaluate your thyroid function, be sure to ask about it.

What happens when I take medication?

Antidepressants increase the amount of the neurotransmitters, such as serotonin, available in the synapse, the space between nerve cells. Whenever symptoms of depression or anxiety appear, there is usually too much or too little of one or more of the neurotransmitters. As shown in the illustration, medication helps the body maintain normal levels of these chemicals, helping to alleviate the symptoms.

How do I know which medication is best?

Deciding on the right medication is a complex process with many variables to consider. Your nurse-practitioner or physician will ask questions about your general health, medications you're currently taking and those you've taken in the past. They may require some laboratory work or other diagnostic/screening tests. The medications used to treat anxiety and depression are distributed throughout the body, not just the brain. For this reason, it is essential that you report which other medications you are taking. Since some medications do not mix well, possible interactions must be considered.

Understanding the Use of Medications

Unlike determining which antibiotic will work best when you have an infection, knowing which psychiatric medication will work for you is not so easy. A trial-and-error approach can be frustrating. If you and your mental health professional decide to try a medication, certain "target symptoms" will be the focus of discussion. As you and your mental health professional monitor the effects of the medication, these symptoms will be evaluated for change. You may also have to test dosages since medications vary in strength. For example, you might take 100 milligrams of one medication but need a dose of 250 milligrams of another

Medication Effects on Nerve Cells

Nerve Cell
Low Serotonin
Depressed Mood

Nerve Cell
Normal Serotonin
Improved Mood

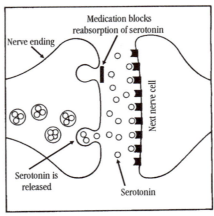

The low serotonin level, shown between nerve cells above, is associated with depression.

The normal level of serotonin between cells is associated with improved mood. Note how the medication blocks the serotonin from being reabsorbed.

medication. This dose variance does not mean that one medication is stronger or better. It is just that their chemical compositions differ. The dose determined for each medication is based on its action.

Side effects are another factor to consider. All medications carry some risk of side effects. For example, aspirin is irritating to the stomachs of some people even as it helps alleviate headache or reduce fever. Some antibiotics have side effects that make them difficult to take. Your prescribing clinician will discuss the temporary side effects that you are likely to experience. These should go away as your body adjusts. You should also be told about more serious or lasting side effects that need to be reported immediately.

Remember: Either take notes when your medication is being described or ask for written information about each one. It is sometimes hard to remember all the information given orally. The psychiatrist or advanced practice nurse may give you a symptom rating sheet to help monitor your symptoms. It is extremely important that you not change the dose or stop taking the medication without talking first to your prescribing clinician.

If you are seeing other health care professionals for other health problems, be sure to tell them about all of your medications. If you buy over-the-counter medications, ask the pharmacist about drug interactions before taking them.

What antidepressants are commonly used?

Several categories of antidepressants are available. Some of the most popular ones are called *selective serotonin reuptake inhibitors*, or SSRIs. They prevent the reabsorption, or reuptake, of serotonin. These drugs are the first choice of clinicians for several reasons. First, they have fewer side effects than some of the older antidepressants. Second, laboratory testing is not required before you can take them.

Selective Serotonin Reuptake Inhibitors (SSRIs)

- Paxil (Paroxetine) 20-60 mg/day
- Prozac (Fluoxetine) 20-80 mg/day
- Luvox (Fluvoxamine) 150-300 mg/day
- Zoloft (Sertraline) 100-200 mg/day

Some people fear becoming addicted to psychiatric medication. However, because these medications help restore your brain chemistry to its normal state, you would not become addicted. Still, you may become accustomed to feeling better with the drug and then feel depressed or anxious when the medication is stopped. This reaction is not the same as addiction, which produces withdrawal symptoms.

There are, however, common side effects from SSRIs; these include difficulty falling asleep, feeling "jittery," problems with sexual functioning, upset stomach, dizziness, and tremors. Most of these side effects are temporary responses to starting the medication. Everyone responds differently to the side effects. It is important to know that many side effects go away after a short time. One exception is a lack of sexual desire and the inability to have an orgasm. If the side effects do not lessen, then the medication may not be the right one for you. Other medications may be given to counteract the side effects so that you do not have to stop taking a medication that is effective for your depression. *Do not stop taking these or any other medications without first talking with your psychiatrist or nurse.* It may be dangerous to stop all at once because doing so may cause abrupt changes in your brain chemistry.

Preliminary evidence shows that women suffering a first-time episode of depression in the postpartum period may respond more quickly and better to SSRIs. The same study also reports that women who started treatment within four weeks postpartum responded more quickly to the medication than did women who started treatment more than four weeks postpartum.

There are also several other newer antidepressants available. The side effects of these medications are varied. Be sure that you know what side effects to look for if any one of these medications is prescribed for you.

Other Antidepressants

- Effexor (Venlafaxine) This medication is often given to the elderly or people sensitive to medication.
- Serzone (Nefazadone) This medication is less likely to cause the nervousness and insomnia of some SSRIs.
- Remeron (Mirtazapine) The newest antidepressant on the market. Its action is different from SSRIs in that it affects both the neurotransmitters serotonin and norepinephrine.
- Wellbutrin (Bupropion) This antidepressant has fewer side effects. It also has less of an effect on sexual functioning than some SSRIs. Although this medication is not new, the dosage recommendations are new.

Tricyclic antidepressants are "older" medications, used when SSRIs and the medications listed above are not effective. The tricyclics are effective, but their side effects make them less tolerable for some. These medications require an EKG if you are over age forty or have a history of heart problems. It also takes four to six weeks before their results are seen. Of the several medications in this category, the most commonly used ones are listed below.

Tricyclic Antidepressants

- Elavil (Amitriptyline) 150-300 mg/day
- Norpramin (Desipramine) 150-300 mg/day
- Pamelor (Nortriptyline) 50-150 mg/day

The most common side effects of tricyclic antidepressants are a dry mouth and constipation. These can be treated by increasing your fluid intake, using a stool softener, or other methods. Additional side effects include dizziness, changes in sex drive, problems urinating, and weight gain.

Another class of medications used to treat depression are *monoamine oxidase inhibitors*, or MAOIs. Although these medications are effective in treating depression, they are usually tried as the last resort when the more common kinds of antidepressants do not work effectively. The MAOIs require dietary changes which make them less popular.

What are commonly used anti-anxiety drugs?

Several medications, including some antidepressants like SSRIs, may help treat both anxiety and depression. But, one of the most common medications used specifically for anxiety is *benzodiazepines*.

Benzodiazepines are minor tranquilizers for panic and severe anxiety. They are to be used with caution and preferably only in short-term intervention because they are potentially addictive. If you have a history of drug abuse, including alcohol, marijuana, nicotine or other substances, be sure to let your health care provider know. A past history of addiction does not mean that you absolutely cannot take benzodiazepines. It just means that they must be used with caution. Benzodiazepines are far less addictive than cocaine, alcohol, barbiturates, or nicotine.

Benzodiazepines differ greatly from antidepressants and other anxiety medications because of their immediate onset and their short duration of effectiveness. As a result, you will need to take these medications several times a day. Another disadvantage of these medications is that tolerance may develop and you may begin to require higher and higher doses. Some people avoid benzodiazepines. Used carefully, however, they can be very helpful in managing the symptoms of panic and severe anxiety.

Another advantage of benzodiazepines is that you can use them as needed rather than having to take them every day. For some people, a regular dose one or more times a day is recommended at the beginning of treatment. As symptoms subside or you gain skill in managing your anxiety, you can sometimes start taking these medications only when you feel anxious. It is very important not to abruptly discontinue these medications if you have been taking a daily dose.

Benzodiazepines useful in treating panic:
- Xanax (alprazolam)
- Klonopin (clonazepam)
- Ativan (lorazepam)

Benzodiazepines useful in treating anxiety:
- Valium (diazepam)

■ Tranxene (clorazepate)
■ Librium (chlordiazepoxide)

The primary side effects you might notice when you start taking benzodiazepines are sleepiness, light-headedness, and sometimes unsteadiness. These side effects should become less of a problem as you continue to take the medication. If they continue, talk to your nurse-practitioner or physician about reducing your dose.

Another drug, BuSpar (Buspirone), is also used to treat anxiety; however it is technically a *nonbenzodiazepine*; it affects different cells in the brain and has no potential for addiction. Side effects for BuSpar include dizziness, headaches, drowsiness, and nausea. You may have to take BuSpar a few weeks before it begins alleviating your anxiety.

Commonly Used Mood Stabilizers

For some women, the mood disorder that emerges during pregnancy or the postpartum state is a kind of depression called bipolar disorder or manic-depressive illness. This illness requires a medication that will even out your mood and will prevent the "highs," or mania, that accompany mood swings. Antidepressants are sometimes given along with these medications because they are primarily effective in stabilizing the mood but may not effectively treat the depression. These medications are sometimes used to help your antidepressant work better.

Mood Stabilizers

■ Eskalith CR, Lithobid (lithium carbonate slow release)
■ Eskalith, lithium carbonate, Lithonate (lithium carbonate)

Property of
Lodi Memorial Library

- Tegretol (carbemazepine)
- Depakote (valproic acid)

The mood stabilizer most commonly prescribed by mental health professionals is *lithium,* a naturally occurring salt which has been in use for many years. If lithium is not helpful, other mood stabilizers are then prescribed. These medications first require extensive laboratory and other screening tests to determine a patient's physical status. All mood stabilizers require ongoing close monitoring and laboratory testing to determine the correct blood level and to monitor potential effects on the liver and kidneys as well as the thyroid.

What is the cost of medication?

The prices of medications vary in different parts of the country and even in different pharmacies in the same town. To find the best price, shop around. You may find it less expensive to use a mail-order pharmacy. One disadvantage of a mail-order pharmacy is that it may be inconvenient to order repeatedly if your dose changes frequently.

Clinicians can sometimes give samples of a medication to see if you can take it or if it is even effective for you. The newer medications are more likely to be available as samples. Ask the person who is prescribing your medication about this option.

Some drug companies have programs for people on low incomes in which they provide medication free or at low cost. These companies usually require the physician or nurse to complete a form and for you to provide proof of your income. If, for budget reasons, you cannot afford these medications, ask your prescribing clinician about this option.

What other kinds of treatments are available?

Support groups are helpful for people with other problems and health disorders, but they are especially important for women with postpartum depression and anxiety because of the new mother's sense of guilt and isolation.

Fortunately, there is a national support organization that was founded by a woman who had postpartum difficulties. Depression after Delivery (DAD) was started in Massachusetts by Nancy Berchtold in 1985. It is now a resource for both health care professionals and women with postpartum mood disorders. Joyce A. Venis, a psychiatric nurse who experienced postpartum depression, is active in DAD. She is a nationally known advocate for women with postpartum complications. She believes "support groups are essential for recovery so that the woman feels validated, supported, and accepted." She recommends that women look for a child-friendly group (with experienced leaders who are knowledgeable about referrals) that can supply you with resources for education and support. Call the national office of DAD (800-944-4773) to see if there is a support group in your area. Dana's story testifies to the helpfulness of a support group:

> *When I became depressed after the birth of my daughter, I got treatment and began to feel better. But it wasn't until I went to a support group for women with postpartum depression that I really felt understood and accepted. It was such a relief to me to find other women who had the same thing happen to them. I wasn't the only one in*

the world! I needed the therapy and medication, but the most important thing that helped me feel better about myself was the support group.

Light therapy is a form of treatment used primarily for people with seasonal affective disorder (SAD), depression thought to be influenced by the amount of light to which we are exposed. There is some evidence that our circadian rhythms influence our mood and that light may play a part in this process. This treatment consists of sitting in front of a 10,000-LUX light for thirty to forty-five minutes daily. Even without looking directly into the light continuously, some people experience antidepressant or mood-stabilizing effects. A new mother named Janice describes how light therapy worked for her:

> *I planned my pregnancy very carefully, because I have had severe depression most of my life. I stopped taking my medication two months before I got pregnant. I was somewhat depressed in the first two trimesters, but in the third I became very depressed, extremely anxious, suicidal, and I could not sleep or eat. I was having major mood swings on a daily basis.*
>
> *I did not want to take any medication, so my psychiatrist suggested I try light therapy. I used the light box three times a week, and it seemed to help. I was still depressed, but it helped me sleep and be less anxious. I was able to delay taking medication until right after delivery.*

A controversial yet relatively safe and very effective treatment for depression is *electroconvulsive therapy* (ECT). This treatment is used for pregnant and postpartum women whose depression has not responded to medication or who cannot take medication. It consists of a series of electrical-shock-induced seizures that take place under anesthesia. Unfortunately, this treatment has a stigma attached to it in most people's minds because of negative depictions of ECT in the media. For example, the movie *One Flew Over the Cuckoo's Nest* depicted a patient undergoing painful shock treatments that seemed to do more harm than good. Modern-day ECT bears no resemblance to the movie version. ECT is given while the patient is sedated with an anesthetic and a muscle relaxant, so no pain is felt. The patient will be sleepy and probably will not even remember what happened for a while after the treatment. ECT is recommended only when all other options are unavailable. A comprehensive review of the use of ECT during pregnancy concludes that ECT during all trimesters in pregnancy was safe and should be considered a valid treatment option. If ECT has been recommended, keep an open mind, seek consultation, and inform yourself about this treatment in more detail.

Hormone therapy is a relatively new treatment that is currently being investigated. The idea behind giving estrogen after delivery is based on the principle that the mood disorders that occur after childbirth are precipitated, not caused, by the abrupt change in estrogen levels after delivery. For women who are at risk for a postpartum mood disorder due to their history of previous problems, this preventive action might help. There are many treatment strategies. It is not possible to exactly predict which one or which combination will work best for you. Be patient and work with your health care professional. Educate yourself about your options and understand why a particular approach is being recommended for you.

7

For Fathers and Families

> *When my wife got depressed just before the baby was born, I was scared, but I thought everything would be okay when the baby got here. No one told me that my wife could have a terrible time being depressed, suicidal, not interested in the baby, and withdrawn from me. I remember living for about a month in terror that my wife would never be the same and that I would have to take care of this baby by myself and cope with the loss of the love of my life.*
>
> *My wife got over her depression. My daughter is almost three, and my wife is wanting another baby. I don't think I can go through that again, not even for another wonderful child.*

Mark's poignant story illustrates the trauma a new father may experience if his wife becomes severely depressed. The unexpected problems frightened Mark so much that he is reluctant to consider having another baby. Postpartum depression drastically affects not only the new mother but also the new father.

Too often, fathers take the "back seat" during pregnancy and after the baby arrives. The focus is on the baby and the mother. As a result, the new father may feel left out and ignored. When the new mother has problems with depression or anxiety, the father's reaction is also often ignored. He is expected to "take care of things" while his wife recovers. There may be little support or education targeted for the man or partner going through such a major crisis.

As a new father, you may be struggling with taking care of both the baby and your wife. You may also be feeling overwhelmed, angry, terrified, incredibly fatigued, or worried. Understand that your feelings are normal.

Why am I so angry?

You may be angry for many reasons. You are under a tremendous amount of stress. The lack of sleep that is affecting your wife so profoundly may also be affecting your own coping skills. You may feel pressured to juggle responsibilities at home and at work. In addition, even though you are trying to be understanding, you may feel that your wife has let you down. After all, no one wants to be solely responsible for an infant. You and your wife had a contract, either implicit or explicit. It may have been that she would take care of the baby while you provided the income, or that you both would work and share in the baby's care. Yet it seems your wife is not living up to her end of the bargain. Be patient and help support her emotionally and practically until she feels better. Only then can she do her part.

If you do not have time off available from work, you may want to consider taking time off under the Family and Medical Leave Act of 1993. You may be eligible to take time to help your wife and baby without endangering your position. There are some restrictions to this policy, though, so be sure to check with your employer's human resources department or benefit administrator.

Unfortunately, there are few support systems designed for fathers or partners. You may not know another husband or partner who has experienced the same problems. Ask others if their wives had problems after delivery. Chances are, you will hear experiences from other fathers that will help you feel less alone.

Lost your wife?

Sometimes men worry that their relationships with their wives will never be the same as before pregnancy. Even under normal circumstances, you would likely find your wife focused on the baby. Keep in mind, though, that she isn't rejecting you. Mother Nature has helped our species survive by providing women with intensely focused mothering behaviors necessary for the helpless infant's survival. As the baby gets older, her intense focus on the baby will lessen.

However, if your wife is having problems with depression or anxiety after childbirth, your concerns may be even greater. Although you may be accustomed to facing problems together, for now you may not be able to rely on her to help you. Despite this loss of her usual coping mechanisms, she will get better. It may be helpful for you to think of the current crisis as a temporary situation. With the treatments available today, you can be optimistic that your wife will once again be your partner. Returning to her old self may take longer than you think it should, but you can help her in many ways.

First of all, listen to her without criticizing or judging. You may not understand what is happening, but neither does she. It will be very helpful to her to be able to talk openly with you. Realize she may feel guilty about her lack of interest in sex at this time. Reassure her that you believe she will soon be like herself again.

Second, participate in her treatment. Educate yourself about postpartum disorders. Don't rely on guess work. Go with your wife to appointments so you can meet the people who are helping her. Understand why a particular treatment has been recommended. Most of all, support your wife in whatever treatment plan she chooses. Even if you aren't comfortable with the therapist or don't like the idea of your wife taking medication, follow her lead. If she feels comfortable with the person or the medication, try not to undermine her efforts by criticizing or disagreeing with the plan of care. Don't ask for details after every therapy session. Let her know you are interested and want to hear only whatever she feels comfortable sharing. Therapy sessions are often very intense, so it may take her awhile to formulate her thoughts.

Third, take on more than your share of responsibility for the baby and the house. Reprioritize your social, athletic, and work commitments to leave you with more time and energy. Taking on this kind of responsibility may be a brand-new experience for which you may not be prepared. But you can do it simply by asking for help and advice from family and friends. Your wife will eventually be able to take on her part, but right now she simply can't.

Fourth, educate both of your extended families about what is happening and how they can help. Criticism or judgmental comments will not help your wife right now. Chances are, family members who are critical do not know about or understand post-partum mood disorders.

These steps to help your wife are going to leave you feeling exhausted, resentful, and overwhelmed. If you need someone to help you at this time, ask your wife's therapist to recommend someone for you. Having someone aware of what you are going through will help you provide better support for your wife.

This difficult time may cause distance between the two of you exactly when you most need to work closely together. If the two of you need marital counseling, arrange for couple's counseling so that you can both air these feelings and renew your partnership, both as a couple and as parents. The following story from thirty-three-year-old Jon illustrates how the marital relationship can be affected by postpartum anxiety:

> *After the baby came, I had to go back to work after taking one week off to be at home. I was feeling this incredible sense of responsibility and felt unprepared to be a father.*
>
> *When my wife started having panic attacks when left alone, I was very angry at her. I thought she was being unreasonable. I felt betrayed by her, like she was leaving me with all the responsibility of the baby, her health, and I had to earn a living! We fought the whole weekend before I was to go back to work. On Sunday, she told me she wanted to kill herself. That scared me so much I called the doctor who delivered the baby. He said, "Sounds like she is having postpartum depression." I was shocked. I didn't know this could happen.*
>
> *I took my wife to see a therapist who explained she was having an anxiety disorder and recommended ther-*

apy and medication. We got a baby-sitter for the day-time, and after about two weeks, my wife was so much better. I met with her therapist to talk about how I was feeling, and that helped. We are back to our good relationship and having a good time with the baby. I am so grateful for the attention paid to our relationship, not just her anxiety.

Jon's feelings about his wife's illness are normal, but choosing the right time and place to express them is important. Just as he experienced relief in talking with someone about how he felt, doing so may prove helpful for you, too. Find someone you feel comfortable with who is knowledgeable about postpartum mood disorders.

I feel responsible.

Even though you both wanted this baby, seeing your wife experience depression or anxiety as a result of having a child may stir up feelings of guilt. Keep in mind that you are not responsible for your wife's condition. But you can help her through her treatment so that you can both enjoy being parents as well as partners.

Should I be worried about safety?

Although most women pose no risk to themselves or their baby, your wife may be so ill that her judgment is impaired. If so, you will need to take action. If she is talking about hurting herself or the baby, take her immediately to the emergency room. Do not leave her alone. Or, if she is agitated, having delusions or hallucinations, seek treatment immediately.

What about the baby?

When my wife had panic attacks and severe anxiety after our son was born, I had to take care of the baby most of the time because she couldn't. I had no clue what I was supposed to do. I had thought I would just play with a baby and love it. I didn't know about feeding, bathing, and the amount of care an infant needs. I got help from several people and I read books, but mostly I learned from taking care of the baby.

This was not my original view of what being a father would be like, but now I wouldn't change it at all. I was even a bit jealous when my wife got better and could take care of him more. But I know I am closer to my son because of the time we spent together.

Ronnie's view of what he was going to do with his baby changed quickly when he had to assume the role of primary caretaker. Our society has gender-based expectations about parenting. Women are supposed to know what to do, while men take a secondary role.

This division of caretaking roles has a historical basis. The traditional father was a breadwinner and a disciplinarian. When household duties were assigned by gender, women took care of the house and the children while men provided the income. When gender roles began to change and women started working more often outside the home, too, their home-based roles did not change as quickly. Even now, research suggests that fathers are typically involved with their children through such activities as sports, while the primary caretaking role is still left to the mother, regardless of whether she is employed outside the home.

It is hard to know for certain how much of this separation of roles is based on tradition. But child care need not be based on the gender of the parent. In reality, some men have stronger nurturing skills than some women, so they make better primary caretakers. If you are having to assume more responsibility for the baby than you thought would be the case, look on this time as an opportunity to experience a connection with your infant that otherwise might not have occurred.

The importance of the infant's attachment to the father is a relatively new idea. Prior to 1970, little research had been done about father-infant or father-child relationships. Since then, though, researchers have discovered that infants attach to the people with whom they come into contact. Attachment to both the mother and father cannot be emphasized enough as a key factor in the infant's development, both physically and mentally.

There is hope.

After ten months, my life is almost like it was before the baby came and my wife got depressed—at least as normal as it can be with a toddler! I no longer wake up scared that things will not be all right. I worry some that my wife will get depressed again. I don't know if we will have another baby.

Patrick's story illustrates the results of successful treatment; his wife is better and his family is back to normal. He will probably always have some worry about his wife, but it no longer dominates his life. Concerns about future pregnancies are very realistic, and may require some serious consideration.

8

Looking Ahead

As you begin to feel better, you will probably find yourself starting to think about the future. Indeed, this response indicates that you *are* feeling better because your perspective is not focused entirely on how you feel right now. But before we discuss the future, let's take a look at where you have been.

As you think about the depression or anxiety that affected you so profoundly, you may find yourself fearful that it will happen again. Most people who have been depressed or affected by severe anxiety dread a recurrence to such an extent that even a slight depression, a bad day, or a period of anxiety may stir up their fears. They may even assume they are back where they started.

But getting better is a gradual process with ups and downs along the way. As you get better, you can anticipate having fewer and fewer bad days, but you will still have some. If you are having a slump after several good days or weeks, do not catastrophize or exaggerate the significance of briefly feeling somewhat like you did before. Juli reacted strongly to increased anxiety and feared she was going to relapse:

> *I had been feeling so good for about three weeks that I thought I was completely cured. Even though my therapist had told me that I would have problems with anxiety again, I secretly told myself I was never going to feel that way again.*
>
> *So, one morning I woke up feeling this ball of anxiety in my stomach, just like I used to. I panicked and called my husband, crying and saying, "It's happening again!" He came home and was very worried. He called my therapist and scheduled an emergency session.*
>
> *By that afternoon I was almost back to normal, but I went to the therapist anyway. I was unrealistic about never having anxiety again. I had to learn to monitor and manage my anxiety. I felt some anger and sadness about having this problem in my life, but fortunately there are medications and people who understand. Now when I have a bad day I make sure I get plenty of sleep, decrease my stress, and ask for help from my husband and friends.*

Juli's unrealistic belief that she was completely over her anxiety and would never have any problems again is not an uncommon reaction. Whenever an illness occurs that profoundly disrupts our lives we want it never to recur. Adjusting to the idea that depression and anxiety may be an ongoing potential problem may take some time.

Now that you are feeling better, you may feel like doing further reading or research about other strategies to help maintain your better mood or calmness. For example, during the early phase of treatment, you may not have felt like going to a support group. Now might be a good time to meet other people with similar problems and learn from them.

I'm better but my family still worries!

As you begin to improve, you may notice that your family shows signs of the stress that has been affecting them. It is not uncommon for families who have been coping well while one member is ill to have a period of time when they fall apart after that family member recovers. You may notice your husband becoming more withdrawn or angry, or your other children may start exhibiting unusual behaviors. This normal readjustment period allows them to express their worry, their anger, and their fear that you will get sick again. Talk about their reactions openly and try to allow them to describe their feelings without trying to fix the situation. Their recovery may be a bit behind yours. They may still be very wary and watchful for signs that you are still ill. Here's what happened in Camilla's family:

> *After I got better, my mother and my husband were still very protective. They wouldn't let me drive very far or take the baby by myself. When I got irritated, they tried to quiet me and tell me not to get upset.*
>
> *Finally I told them that I was better and that they needed to loosen up. They both cried and said they were so worried about me that they didn't want me to get depressed again. My therapist suggested that I tell them they don't need to worry so much because I have others who will help me monitor how I am feeling. This talk helped a lot. Now they treat me normally, not like an invalid.*

What do I tell people?

Now that you are out and about more, telling friends and family about your depression or anxiety may be stressful. During the acute or severe part of your illness, your focus was on feeling better and getting treatment. Now that you are feeling better, it is up to you to decide how much to share and with whom you should share your experiences.

Will it happen again if I have another baby?

If you experienced depression or anxiety during a previous pregnancy, you are at risk of another occurrence. If you find yourself feeling as you did during your previous pregnancy, seek help immediately. Lorraine, a twenty-nine-year-old, describes her anxiety during three pregnancies:

> *I had my first episode of anxiety during my first pregnancy when I was about ten weeks pregnant. I couldn't sleep. I thought I was dying at times. My doctor referred me to a therapist who was very helpful.*
>
> *After the baby came, I thought the panic might come back, but it didn't. However, the panic did return during my next two pregnancies. The last time, I had to use medication to help me control the symptoms during the last trimester. I have not had any problems except when I was pregnant.*

Even though you may be at risk for another past postpartum disorder, your previous experience does not absolutely mean you will have trouble again. Each pregnancy is different. Your mind and body are different now. And, now that you have had some experience with treatment, keep in mind that if you do become depressed or anxious again, seeking early treatment is better than trying to ride it out on your own. In addition to treatment, there are many things you can do yourself. Take care of yourself and try to stay physically healthy: get enough sleep, eat nutritious meals, and exercise. Yes, it isn't easy if you have young children, but it is not impossible. Make sure that your social needs are met. Don't focus all of your energy on your family. You need some space for your own interests and time alone or with your friends. Doing so does not mean that you are being selfish. Don't say yes to everyone else and no to yourself. A major part of taking care of ourselves is to be sure that we have some fun in our own lives. What do you do for fun? If the only answer you have is collapsing in front of the TV after putting your children to bed, then perhaps you need to develop an outlet for yourself.

Minimize the stress in your life. Your recovery may take longer than you think. Perhaps you can put off that remodeling job or the move to a bigger house for a while. If you have gone back to work, perhaps you can consciously make an effort not to overextend yourself. For many young families, finances are a major source of stress. Perhaps a consultation with a financial planner can help ease your stress about money.

Nurture your relationships. Connections with other people are vital to both our physical and mental health. To prosper and grow, our relationships need careful attention. Don't neglect the relationship with your husband. Be sure to spend time alone as a couple on "dates" so that you can reconnect as adults who once fell in love, when it was just the two of you. You need to nurture this relationship now because someday it will be just the two of you again, and you don't want to be strangers.

Watch out for early warning signs. By now you probably recognize the signs that you are getting anxious or depressed. Perhaps you are not sleeping well for several weeks, or sleeping too much. Maybe you notice that you don't want to leave the house. Do you notice that you feel irritable and get angry over small issues? Often, recognizing early signs and paying attention to them can head off another episode. If the symptoms persist, call your therapist. Paying attention to the balance in your life and correcting any "tilts" will help. Remember that achieving balance is a process. If you get out of balance, it doesn't mean you are back to where you started. It just means that you need to do whatever is necessary to help regain your equilibrium.

If you decide to have another child, it may be helpful to wait at least two years so that you do not have more than one infant at the same time. Be sure to tell all of your caregivers about your previous episode of postpartum depression or anxiety. Talk with your therapist early in your pregnancy about a treatment plan in case you develop symptoms again. Sometimes medication may be started immediately after delivery to ward off an episode of depression. Many women have found this very effective.

What about taking medications during pregnancy?

During the time of conception and your first missed period, the placenta has not yet developed, so the likelihood of the medication affecting your baby is small. However, after the first missed period, the placenta forms, so medication can reach the baby. Don't wait for a pregnancy test to talk with your physician about medications if you have any suspicions.

As a general rule, most medications are withheld during pregnancy whenever possible, particularly during the first trimester. After this time the baby's vital organs have formed, and the risk is less. However, the safety of the mother is also considered. This is a difficult decision because both the risks and benefits must be considered. Talk to your caregivers about medications. Most of the time what they will tell you is that the risk is unknown because there have not been many studies done to determine risk. Most of what we know comes from case reports and animal studies. Based on what is known, the Food and Drug Administration does list risk categories for drugs for use during pregnancy.

Enjoy the journey ahead...

Today is an exciting time to become a mother. Never before in history have we had access to such advanced medical technology—technology that helps insure the health and well-being of both mother and child. Whether a mother's needs are physical or emotional, help is available.

Seek the support of knowledgeable professionals. There is no reason to suffer in silence and in shame. In fact, early intervention while you are pregnant is essential to both your health and your baby's health. You can find considerable relief in working with an informed therapist. The very act of talking about what you are feeling often helps. Don't fall prey to the common misconception that pregnancy or motherhood is always a time of bliss. You deserve to feel good about this important phase of your life. Understand that any depression or anxiety now is just a small part of the process. With proper treatment, you can enjoy becoming a mother.

Appendix / Resources

Depression After Delivery
   P.O. Box 1282
   Morrisville, PA 19067
   800-944-4773 (information packet)

La Leche League (www.lalecheleague.com)
   1400 N. Meacham
   Schaumburg, IL 60168
   800-525-3243
   847-455-7730 (central time)

Marcé Society
   c/o Michael O'Hara
   Department of Psychology
   University of Iowa
   Iowa City, IA 52242
   319-335-2405

Postpartum Support International
   927 N. Kellogg Avenue
   Santa Barbara, CA 93111
   805-967-7636

Anxiety Disorders Association of America
6000 Executive Blvd., Suite 513
Rockville, MD 20852-3801
310-231-8368

Freedom from Fear
308 Seaview Avenue
State Island, NY 10305
718-351-1717

National Depressive and Manic-Depressive Association
730 Franklin, Suite 501
Chicago, IL 60610
312-642-0049

Obsessive Compulsive Foundation
P.O. Box 70
Milford CT 06460-0070
203-878-5669

Office of Scientific Information
National Institute of Mental Health
5600 Fishers Lane, Room 7C-02
Rockville, MD 20857
301-443-4513

Professional Organizations

DOULAS Of North America
1100 23rd Avenue East
Seattle, WA 98112
206-324-5440

American Nurses Association
    600 Maryland Ave SW, Suite 100 West
    Washington, DC 20024
    202-651-7000

American Psychiatric Association
    1400 K Street
    Washington, DC 20005
    202-682-6000

American Psychiatric Nurses Association
    1200 19th Street NW, Suite 300
    Washington, DC 20036
    202-857-1133

American Psychological Association
    750 First Street NW
    Washington, DC 20002
    202-336-5500

National Association of Cognitive-Behavioral Therapists
    P.O. Box 2195
    Weirton, WV 26002
    800-853-1135

National Association Of Social Workers
    750 First Street NE, Suite 700
    Washington, DC 20002
    800-638-8799

Bibliography

Chapter 1

Barnett, Robert, MD. Interview with author. August 2, 1996.

Buist, A. & B. Barnett. 1995. Childhood sexual abuse: a risk factor for postpartum depression. *Australian and New Zealand Journal of Psychiatry.* 29:4.

Creasy, R.K. & R. Resnik. 1994. *Maternal-fetal medicine: Principles and practice.* Philadelphia: W.B. Saunders.

Dix, C. 1985 *The new mother syndrome.* New York: Pocket Books.

Hamilton, J.A., & P.N. Harberger, eds. 1992. *Postpartum psychiatric illness: A picture puzzle.* Philadelphia: University of Pennsylvania Press.

Iles, S., D. Gath, & H. Kennerley. 1989. Maternity blues: A comparison between post-operative women and post-natal women. *British Journal of Psychiatry.* 155:363-366.

Kendall, R.E., J.C. Chalmers, & C. Platz. 1987. Epidemiology of puerperal psychoses. *British Journal of Psychiatry.* 150:662-673.

Morrison, Grace, MD. Interview with author. August 6, 1996.

O'Hara, M.W., J.A. Schlechte, D.A. Lewis, & E.J. Wright. 1991. Prospective study of postpartum blues: Biologic and psychosocial factors. *Archives of General Psychiatry.* 48:801-806.

Schmidt, Manya, CNM, ARNP. Interview with author. August 16, 1996.

Sichel, D. Lecture given at American Psychiatric Association meeting, New York, New York, May 5, 1996.

Statistical Abstract of the United States. 1994. United States Department of Commerce: Washington, D.C.

The World Almanac and Book of Facts. 1996. Mahwah, New Jersey: World Almanac Books.

Chapter 2

Kennerly, H. & D. Gath. 1989. Maternity blues: Associations with obstetric, psychological and psychiatric factors. *British Journal of Psychiatry.* 155:367-373.

O'Hara, M.W., et al. eds. 1995. *Psychological aspects of women's reproductive health.* New York: Springer.

Chapter 3

American Psychiatric Association. 1994. *Diagnostic and statistical manual of mental disorders.* 4th ed. Washington, D.C.: American Psychiatric Books.

Bibliography

Andrews, G. et al. 1994. *The treatment of anxiety disorders: Clinician's guide and patient manuals.* Cambridge, U.K.: Cambridge University Press.

Engler, J. & D. Goleman. 1992. *The consumer's guide to psychotherapy.* New York: Simon & Schuster.

Misri, S. 1995. *Shouldn't I be happy: Emotional problems of pregnant and postpartum women.* New York: Free Press.

Chapter 4

American Psychiatric Association. 1994. *Diagnostic and statistical manual of mental disorders.* 4th ed. Washington, D.C.: American Psychiatric Association.

Beck, C.T. 1995. The effects of postpartum depression on maternal-infant interaction: A meta-analysis. *Nursing Research.* 44:5.

Hamilton, J.A. & P.N. Harberger. eds. 1992. *Postpartum psychiatric illness: A picture puzzle.* Philadelphia: University of Pennsylvania Press.

Hay, D.F., & R. Kumar. 1995. Interpreting the effects of mother's post-natal depression on children's intelligence: A critique and re-analysis. *Child Psychiatry and Human Development.* 25 (3):165-181.

Healy, B. 1995. *A new prescription for women's health: Getting the best medical care in a man's world.* New York: Penguin.

Jack, D.C. 1991. *Silencing the self: Women and depression.* Cambridge, Mass: Harvard University Press.

Maldonado, M. M.D. Interview with author. May 6, 1996.

McGrath, E. ed. 1990. *Women and depression.* Washington, D.C.: American Psychological Association.

O'Hara, M.W. et al. eds. 1995. *Psychological aspects of women's reproductive health.* New York: Springer Publishing.

Paffenbarger, R.S. 1982. Epidemiological aspects of mental illness associated with childbearing. I.F. Brockington & R. Kumar, eds. *Motherhood and mental illness.* New York: Grune and Stratton.

Papolos, D., & J. 3d ed. 1997. *Overcoming depression.* New York: Harper Perennial. An excellent book about depression, particularly bipolar illness.

Parry, B.L. 1989. Reproductive Factors Affecting the Course of Affective Illness in Women. *Psychiatric Clinics of North America.* 12.1: 207-220.

Pauliekhoff, B. 1992. Toward the diagnosis of postpartum psychotic depression. Hamilton, J.A. & P.N. Harberger, eds. *Postpartum psychiatric illness: A picture puzzle.* Philadelphia: University of Pennsylvania Press.

Sichel, D.A., et al. 1995. Prophylactic estrogen in recurrent postpartum affective disorder. *Biological Psychiatry.* 38:814-818.

Bibliography

Stern, D.N. 1985. *The interpersonal world of the infant.* New York: Basic Books.

Stowe, Z.N., et al. 1995. Sertraline in the treatment of women with postpartum major depression. *Depression.* 3:49-55.

Wieck, A. et al. 1991. Increased sensitivity of dopamine receptors and recurrence of affective psychosis after childbirth. *British Medical Journal.* 303 (6803):613-616.

Chapter 5

Andrews, G. et al. 1994. *The treatment of anxiety disorders: Clinician's guide and patient manuals.* New York: Cambridge University Press.

Antonuccio, D.O., W.G. Danton, & G.Y. DeNelsky. 1995. Psychotherapy versus medication for depression: Challenging the conventional wisdom with data. *Professional Psychology: Research and Practice.* 26 (6):574-585.

Engler, J. & D. Goleman. 1992. *The consumer's guide to psychotherapy.* New York: Fireside Books.

Meager, I. & J. Milgrom. 1996. Group treatment for postpartum depression: A pilot study. *Australian and New Zealand Journal of Psychiatry.* 30:852-860.

Mental health: Does therapy help? *Consumer Reports.* November, 1995.

Miller, I. W., & G.I. Keitner. 1996. Combined medication and psychotherapy in the treatment of chronic mood disorders. *The Psychiatric Clinics of North America.* 19 (1):151-169.

Chapter 6

Ferrill, M.J., W.A. Kehoe, & J.J. Jacism. 1992. ECT during pregnancy: Physiologic and pharmacologic considerations. *Convulsive Therapy.* 8 (3):186-200.

Hyman, S.E. et al. 1995. *Handbook of Psychiatric Drug Therapy.* 3d Ed. New York: Little, Brown.

McEwen, B.S. 1996. How the brain works. *Women's Health Digest.* 2 (1):33-36.

Palmer, L.K. 1995. Effects of a walking program on attributional style, depression, and self-esteem in women. *Perceptual and Motor Skills.* 81:891-898.

Richelson, E. 1994. Pharmacology of antidepressants—Characteristics of the ideal drug. *Mayo Clinic Proceedings.* 69:1069-1081.

Sichel, D.A., et al. 1995. Prophylactic estrogen in recurrent postpartum affective disorder. *Biological Psychiatry.* 38:814-818.

Stowe, Z.N., J. Casserella, J. Landry, & C.B. Nemeroll. 1995. Sertraline in the treatment of women with postpartum major depression. *Depression.* 3:49-55.

Bibliography

Thayer, R.E., et al. 1994. Self-regulation of mood: Strategies for changing a bad mood, raising energy and reducing tension. *Journal of Personality and Social Psychology.* 67 (5):910-925.

Venis, Joyce, R.N. Communication with author. June 15, 1997.

Chapter 7

Lamb, M.E. ed. 1997 *The role of the father in child development.* 3d ed. New York: John Wiley.

Public Law 103-3. *United States Statutes at Large.* vol. 107, part 1. Washington D.C.: United States Government Printing Office.

Chapter 8

Bibring, G.L. et al. 1961. A study of the psychological processes in pregnancy and of the earliest mother-child relationship. *The psychoanalytic study of the child.* 15:9-24.

Briggs, G.G., R.K. Freeman, & S.J. Yaffe. 1990. *Drugs in pregnancy and lactation.* 3d. ed. Williams and Wilkins: Baltimore, MD.

Cohen, L.S. et al. 1996. Course of panic disorder during pregnancy and the puerperium: A preliminary study. *Biological Psychiatry.* 39:950-954.

Paffenbarger, R.S. 1982. The epidemiological aspects of mental illness associated with childbearing. Brockington, I.F. and R. Kumar. eds. *Motherhood and mental illness.* Grune & Stratton: New York.

Index

About the Author

L inda Sebastian has been a psychiatric nurse for twenty-five years. As an Advanced Registered Nurse Practitioner, she provides outpatient therapy and medication management. Ms. Sebastian served as the Director of the Women's Program at the Menninger Foundation, Topeka, Kansas, from 1994 to 1998. The program was recognized nationally for its treatment of depression in women. As part of the program, Ms. Sebastian developed the perinatal psychiatric disorders program and has been active in educating professionals about postpartum depression and anxiety.

Ms. Sebastian received a master's degree in psychiatric nursing from Kansas University in 1982. She graduated from the Wesley School of Nursing in Wichita, Kansas, in 1972, and earned a bachelor's degree in psychology from Kansas University in 1976. Ms. Sebastian has received national certification from the American Nurses Credentialing Center and the National Association of Cognitive-Behavioral Therapists.

Ms. Sebastian is the author of numerous professional journal articles, and is active in professional organizations; she has been a featured speaker in the United States and China. Ms. Sebastian lives in Topeka, Kansas, with her husband and two children.